Men's Sexual Health

How to use your pelvic floor muscles in everyday activities?

Judith Moricz

Health Educator

The creator of the IWT® Pelvic Floor Exercises

Intimate Wellness Training for men - IWT®

Men's Sexual Health

For further information, please contact:

Judith Moricz

jmpublichealthexpert@gmail.com

Disclaimer

The information provided in this book is meant for informational and educational use only. It is not intended to replace guidance or care of a medical professional. If you believe you have symptoms, mentioned in this book or any other illness, please consult with the appropriate health care professional for specific diagnosis and treatment. The author is not liable for the misuse or misinterpretation of the information provided in this book.

Sexual Health

Goes beyond

Physical Health…

Contents of the book

INTRODUCTION

Everybody would like to be healthy. However, the question is if one will be ready to make efforts to avoid the causes of illness to reach that aim.

The normal condition of man is being healthy. The modern, civilized way of living that differs from the natural, results in an unnatural physiological state – this is what we call illness. Unfortunately, a decisive part of mankind has become symptom-free Homo Patient instead of Homo Sapiens. It is a mistake to think that if one has neither complaint nor pain it means he is healthy.

You often hear about the importance of physical health and mental health, but feeling confident about your sexual health also is very important. Sexual health help us to figuring out what are our values, determine our self-image and self-esteem, affects our emotional state and the quality of our personal relationships. In both, men and women, the pelvic floor is an active sexual organ. However, its role in sexual dysfunction is often underestimated. For many people, the pelvic floor does not work as well as it should.

Sexual health covers not only medical or reproductive issues but all aspects of sex education such as disease prevention, intimate hygiene, practicing safer sex to prevent Sexually Transmitted Infections (STIs), to learn about contraception methods, sexual behavior and sexual attitudes. That is why it is essential to be well informed about all aspects of sexual health.

The development of a disease is generally a long process – lasting even for decades on occasions. Health is not a self-forming or durably existing state; we must do something to preserve it day after day! It is our own duty and responsibility to preserve our health. Most people are not aware of that. They are dread of illness, and if they still get ill, they are willing to think that they are the victims of a random misfortune. Let's not shift the responsibility and blame others or fate, let us not expect drugs or operations to keep us healthy, but rather take an active part in preserving and regaining our health.

As far as I see, a gradually increasing number of people think it necessary and important to take their health in their own hands. Accordingly, it is very important to learn the ways and methods of avoiding or preventing illness and the natural curing methods and opportunities. Those methods that promise a quick and easy recovery in a way that one should nearly do nothing for success, always offer a temporary solution only.

As the saying goes, it is not the disease that is incurable, but the patient. It all depends on the degree the person involved is willing to explore and face the physical-mental causes of his illness, then on the volume of energy and time he is ready to spend in order to eliminate or avoid the inducing factors. Who is willing to make efforts as concerns both his lifestyle and the conscious changing of his positive mental attitude, may indisputably cherish the hope for recovery! I wish you all success and persistence to reach that goal!

I hope my written work contains valuable advices for anyone who comes to read it, by following which he will be able to live a more healthy and happy life!

This Book contains general suggestions, so the methods described therein cannot replace professional diagnosis and therapy.

THE PELVIC FLOOR

Why we neglect our perineal muscles? In general, we only care for those muscles that take part in the shaping of our body or serve the preservation of our right posture, such as the abdominal muscles, the gluteal, biceps or dorsal etc. muscles. We do not even think of the muscles of the pelvic floor, we do not miss their training as long as they completely fulfill their function. Another reason is that muscular strength diminishing, muscular atrophy at the beginning do not cause characteristic signs and symptoms, as they occur slowly and insidiously. We live together with the symptoms and do not even notice that they are part of our everyday life. The muscular tonus of the neglected pelvic floor muscles gradually diminishes as time passes, the muscles becomes more and more inflexible, and their contractility and strength gets weaker. This may occur at any age. If we do not exercise these interior PC-muscles regularly, the slackening of their strength may start already at young age. If pelvic floor muscles lose their strength, complaints involving urinary or fecal incontinence or different sexual problems may occur.

Sexual Health does not exist without strong pelvic floor muscles!

In order to know how to do pelvic floor (Kegel) exercises correctly, you need to know where your pelvic floor muscles are.

Let 'see where the perineal muscles are?

The simplest definition of the perineum is; the part of the body that sits on the bicycle seat. This is the "intimate part" of our body that greatly influences the voluntary control over defecation and urination. The same muscles support the erection just like the voluntary control over ejaculation in males. Orgasms feel bigger and stronger when pelvic floor muscles are strong. Strong and controlled pelvic floor muscles can seriously improve your sex life! We might think that the bottom of the pelvis is composed of several large and strong muscles, but it is not so. Pelvic floor muscles compared to other muscles in our body are so small and tiny, that the thickness and the entire surface area does not exceed the size of the palm of our hand.

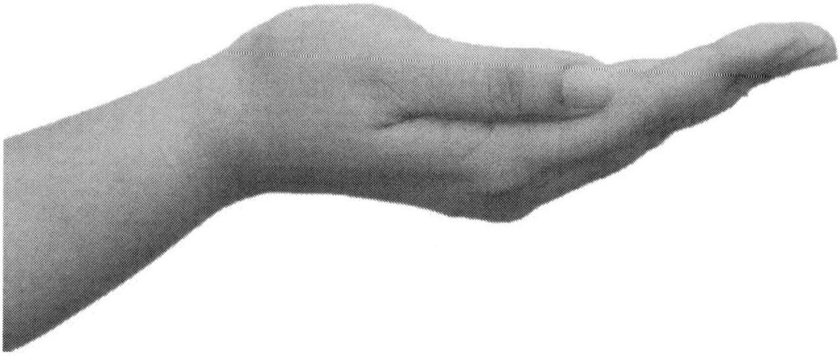

Precisely these muscles are located between the pubic bone anteriorly and the Coccyx (tail-) bone posteriorly. The pelvic floor is a complex, integrated, multilayer system that provides active and passive support.

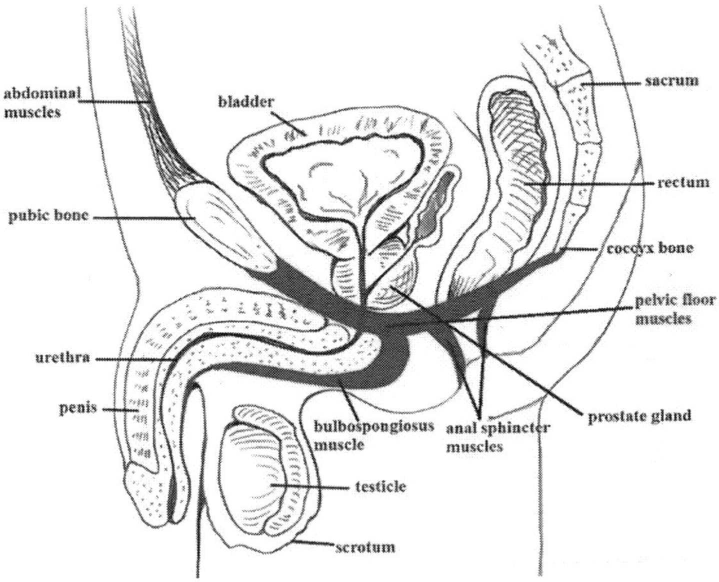

The pelvic floor has three layers: internal - middle and external called superficial layer. In case of men, there are two openings through the pelvic floor: one to allow the urethra to pass through on its way from the bladder to the penis and the other at the anus. The pelvic floor muscles normally wrap quite firmly around these holes to help keep the passages shut. There is also an extra circular muscle around the anus (the external and internal anal sphincter) and around the urethra (the external and internal urethral sphincter). The internal sphincter muscles (both urethral and anal) are involuntary muscles, which should be closed at all times, except when you are actually trying to open your bowels or to urinate. Their function normally depends on the "sympathetic" nervous system, which governs the automatic functions; they will open only after the evacuation or urination reflex. The outer rings of muscles are the external sphincters, which are voluntary muscles, which you can tighten up to close them more firmly if you have diarrhea or urgency to urinate. Both sphincter muscles wrap right around the anus and urethra. Either or both of these sphincter muscles (internal or external – anal/ urethral) can become weak at any age. Dysfunction in pelvic floor muscles is increasingly common in men. This may be because of a sedentary lifestyle or from regular constipation and straining or general wear and tear or during radical prostatectomy surgery. Sometimes there is no obvious reason why. If you have weak pelvic floor muscles you may leak urine, gas or solid stools or you may have erection problems.

The perineal muscles in men are less sunken and more strained. The part of the superficial perineal muscles - that in the case of women surrounding the urethral and vaginal orifice - in males is an attached part and supports from below the initial part of the penis (root of the penis). In men, the function of these muscles is visible, so having an obvious signal when their perineal muscles are moving, they are able to learn quickly the pelvic floor exercises and to move them voluntarily. The muscles of the pelvic floor are the same for both men and women. The difference is in their position because of gender diversity and the size of the male pelvis and reproductive organs.

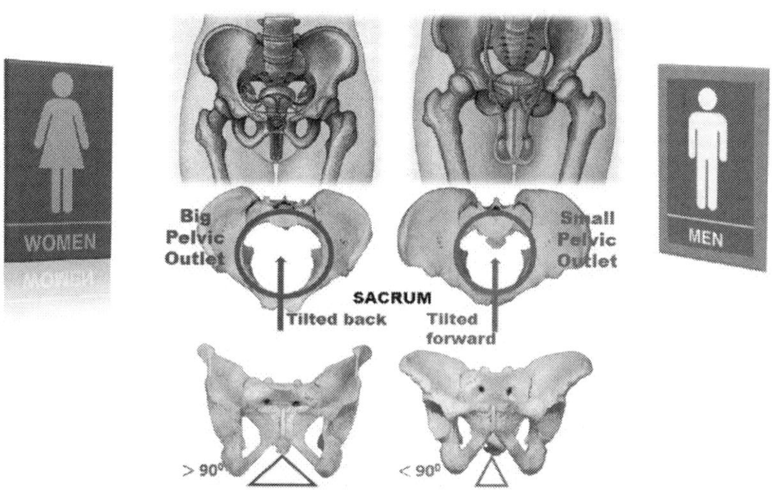

What are the functions of the pelvic floor?

In animals – as a consequence of their body position – slightly any burden is loaded on the muscles closing the pelvis, since the weight of their interior organs is held by the strong abdominal musculature. During phylogenesis, as a result of bipedal movement this function was shifted on the muscles of the pelvic floor.

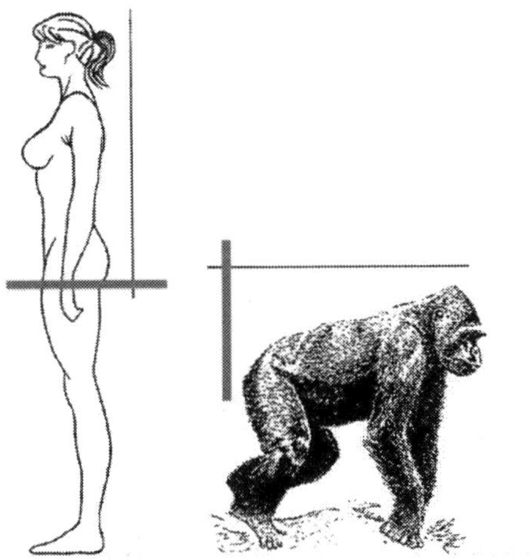

These muscles are stretched out on the bottom of the pelvis like a flexible trampoline and hold the organs to be found above them against the permanent gravitational power. The tight and flexible "trampoline" resists another power, too, which is generated by the development of the increasing pressure in the abdominal cavity. Through the orifices on the pelvic floor, the urethra and the rectum open to the outside world.

The function of the pelvic floor is complex, to close the pelvic exit and underpin the organs of the pelvis minor thereby. By way of its closing function it opens-closes or keeps closed the opening (sphincters) of the urethra and the anus - according to the actual need. The same muscles are responsible for the angle and quality of erection in males. There are two types of striated muscle fibers: they consist of muscular fibers able to either fast or slow contraction. This is the case with the musculature of the pelvic floor. The quickly contracting fibers cause the contractions accompanied by maximum-intensity sudden exertion. The slow fibers take part in the less-intense, but longer-term work. This can be easily understood if we think what happens on sneezing: the perineal muscles are suddenly contracted; the fast-twitch muscle fibers are activated preventing thereby the urinary discharge. However, when the bladder is filled with urine, the muscular work needed to retain urination is carried out – with persistent tension – by the slow twitch muscle fibers. In training the pelvic floor, both types of muscle fibers should be strengthened.

But what factors induce weakening of the pelvic floor?

On the one hand, our perineal muscles are exposed to extreme load since we live in human civilization as bipeds. The unloaded, nearly perpendicular perineal musculature took up a horizontal position when we evolved our two-legged upright walking style whereby the weight of our internal organs is gradually shifted on it. This weight – in the case of weakened or damaged pelvic floor muscles by various factors – is just enough to cause physical problems and early symptoms (like urine leakage or difficulty achieving or maintaining an erection) by which will be sooner or later experienced by everyone. On the other hand, we have several bad everyday habits by which we continuously load the muscles of the pelvic floor. These are, for example: we are able to sit on them for hours (that is we continuously compress the pelvic floor muscles from below and stiffen them). In addition to that, we sit in an improper, curved posture (that is we exert a pressure from above on the weak and stiffened perineal muscles).

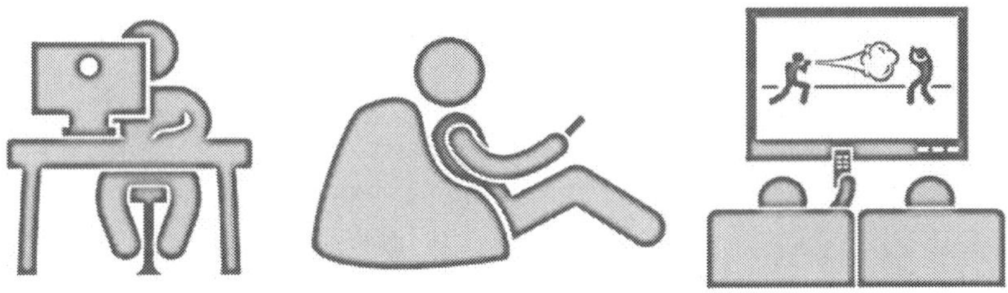

We discharge the waste material leaving our body (urine, stool) with an inadequate technique, we have no idea how could we relieve the burden on our bladder when getting up in the morning for example, we often carry heavy loads and practice sports with improper technique, too. With our many bad everyday habits, we involuntarily weaken the intimate muscles continuously, while we expect our sphincters to carry out their functions perfectly.

Various risk factors can play a role in the development of Pelvic Floor Symptoms (urinary, bowel and sexual functions), but these involve a predisposition only and do not cause incontinence in themselves. Continence problems present themselves only if several risk factors occur at the same time or if the mechanism of urination gets damaged at any stage or if the muscles of the pelvic floor are for some reason durably exposed to an extraordinary load.

Let us enroll some of the risk factors!

Defecation and urination regularly involving strong abdominal pressure are harmful. Those, who every day has to make durable efforts and exertion to discharge stool with abdominal press, overloading their pelvic floor muscles, may endure serious perineal damage.

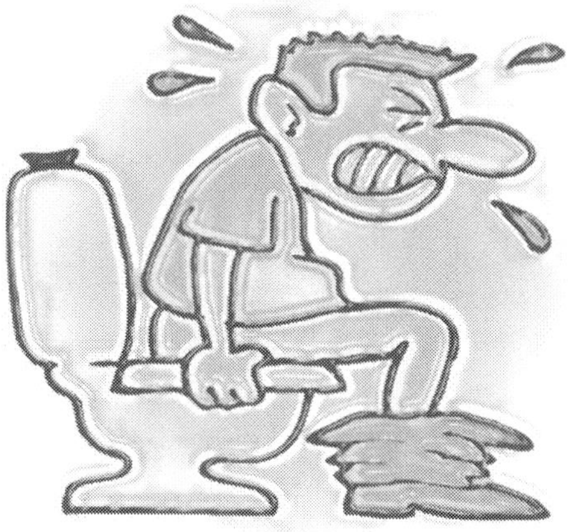

Bad posture, stretching the supporting ligaments of the lower abdominal organs and constricting the blood circulation of the perineum.

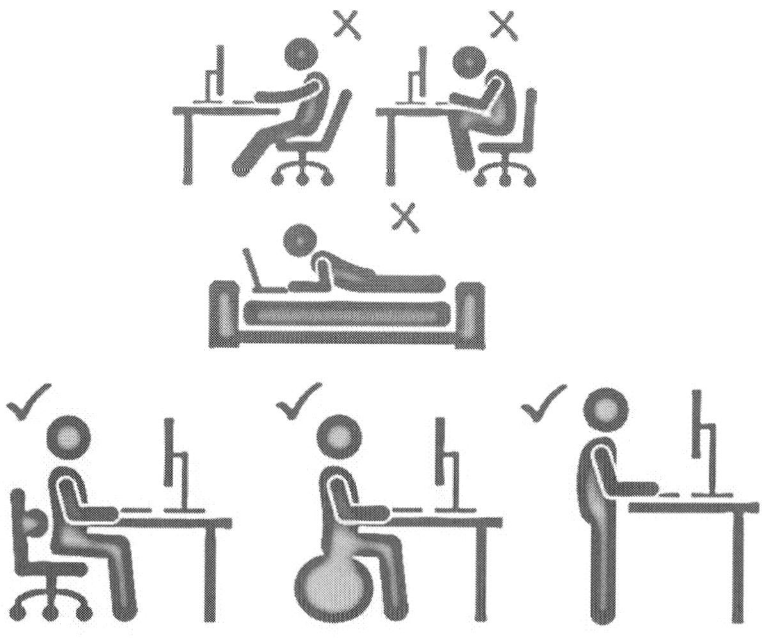

Another risk factor is ***obesity***. An overweight exceeding 10 kg loads an extra burden on the lower abdominal organs, thus the heavier visceral organs load a stronger stress on the pelvic floor muscles.

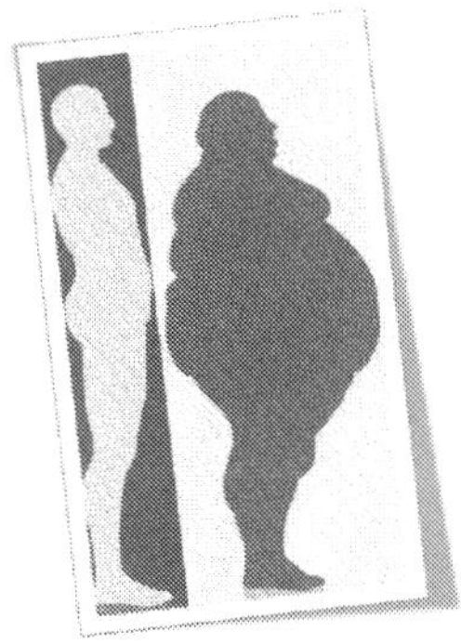

In the case of ***diseases, involving coughing and sneezing***, the strong shaking effect occurring in the pelvis, overloads the ligaments holding the pelvic organs and the muscles of the pelvic floor.

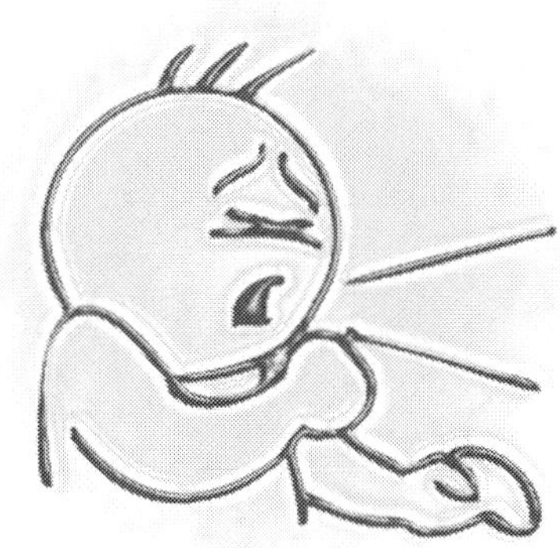

As in every closed space, a certain pressure is present in the abdominal cavity, which is also subject to the rules of physics. The volume of this pressure is changing all the time: as per the rhythm of breathing, following the stretching of the abdominal muscles, or even according to the changes of the bodily position. On coughing, sneezing or laughing the diaphragm and the abdominal muscles gets quickly tightened together, resulting in a considerable and sudden increase in pressure. If the muscles of the pelvic floor are strong enough and work properly, that is able to resist and compensate the increased abdominal pressure occurring in the abdominal cavity from time to time, they will also be able to underpin the abdominal organs and keep the sphincters properly closed. If, however, the pelvic floor muscles are weakened and lowered, being exposed to the burden caused by the increased pressure in this state, it will be unable to prevent the discharge of drops of urine. The more frequent the growth of pressure in the abdomen, the stronger the burden loaded on the pelvic floor and the greater the risk of incontinence is.

The hard physical work – with frequent motions involving pushing, lifting, pulling – requiring great exertion may result in the lengthening of the supporting ligaments of the pelvic organs.

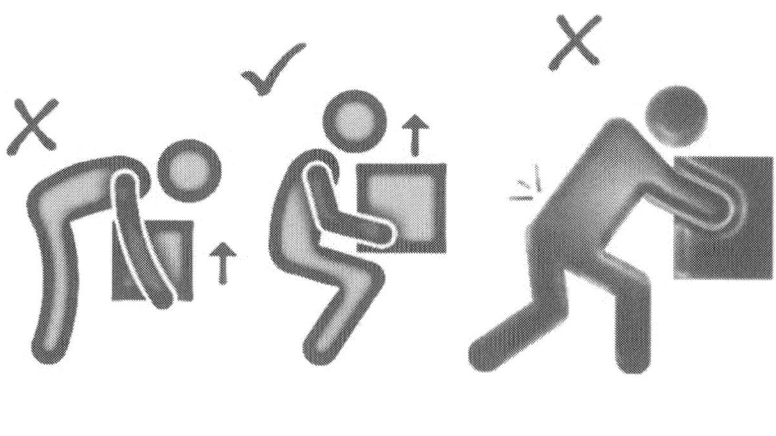

The work done by those who lift heavy objects and carry heavy loads for hours, keeping their abdominal muscles work all the time, increasing thereby the pressure in their abdominal cavity. This may have a very negative influence on the lower abdominal organs.

Improperly exercised fitness or sport activities, disregarding the vulnerability of the pelvic floor. This may involve skipping, hopping or weight-training exercises carried out in a perpendicular trunk position.

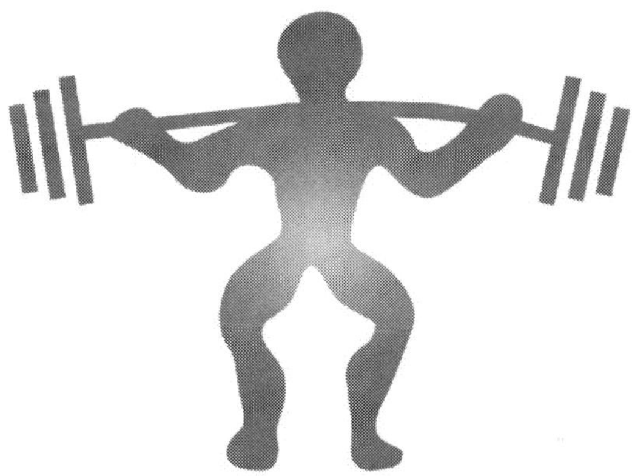

Working hard for their "health", these people do not care how much harm their interior muscles are done. Making these mistakes in a steady and persistent way, we may suffer damages without even noticing anything.

In the case of ***durable or frequently occurring stressful situations*** the muscles of the pelvic floor becomes more tense, their blood vessels narrow down, which results in insufficient blood circulation and nutrition for proper muscle function.

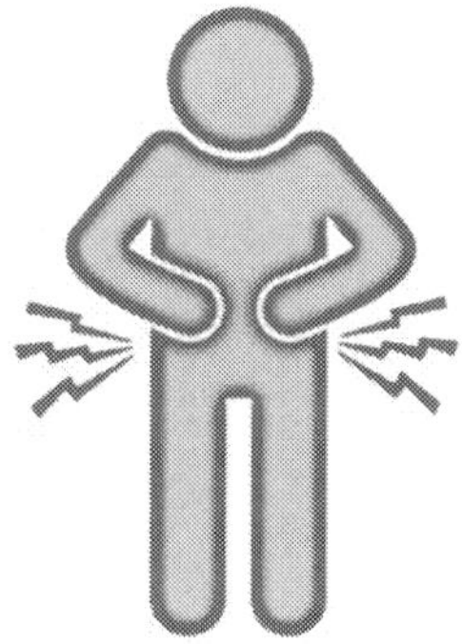

Nicotine is a potent vasoconstrictor therefore, as a consequence of smoking the perineal blood vessels narrow down, entailing poorer blood circulation, not to mention strong coughing that also burdens the pelvic floor muscles.

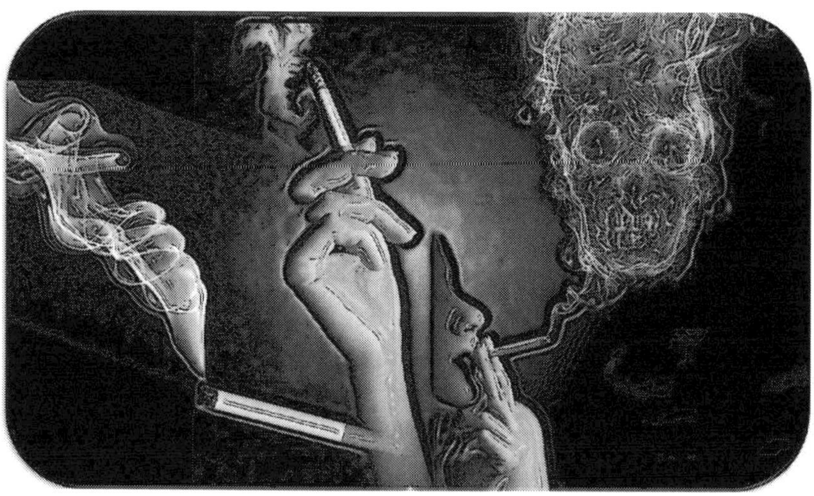

In the case of ***frequent inflammation of the pelvic region*** (for example prostatitis – inflammation of the prostate), the tone of the tissues involved in the abnormality diminishes.

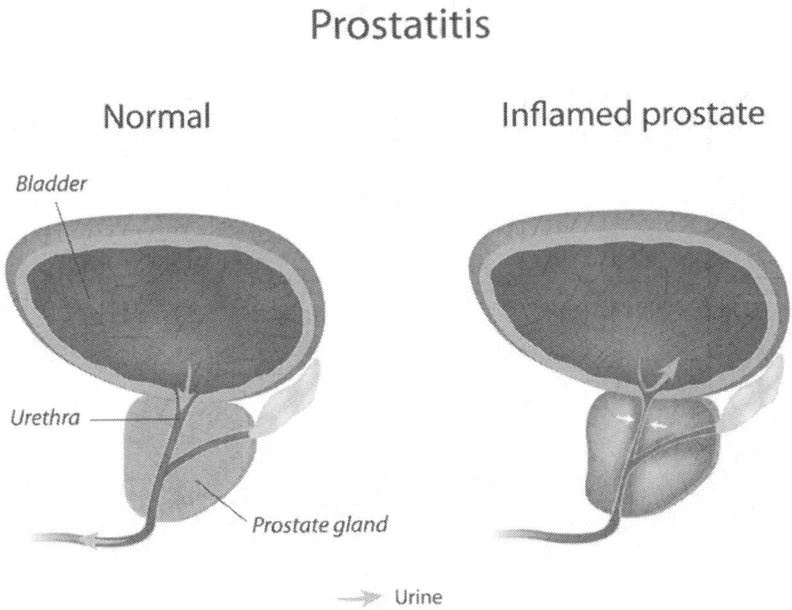

A frequent predisposing factor to intimate problems is the ***inappropriate, inflexible connective tissue substance***. This may be caused – among others – by its weak congenital structure, but the progress of time may also have a negative effect on its condition. In the case of weak connective tissue, the pelvic floor can be easily damaged even by average loading. The tissues, the supporting ligaments are less resistant, requiring higher protection accordingly. It is not only the congenital factors and the natural process of aging that have an influence on the condition of the connective tissue and the muscles, but hormones, too.

Any surgery affecting the pelvis minor or lower abdominal organs may involve the risk of muscular or nerve injury, which will inhibit urinary continence.

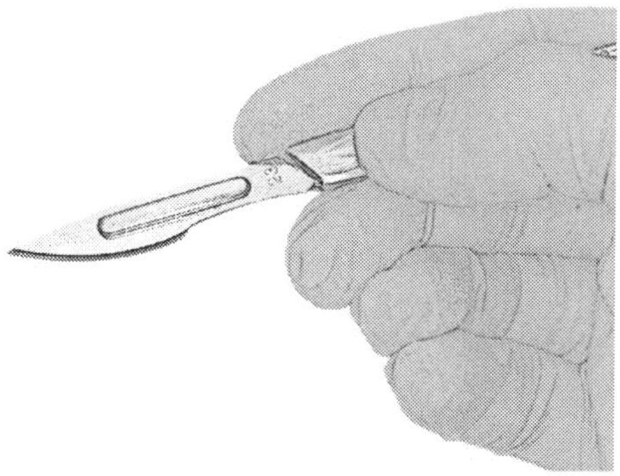

Congestion caused by inadequate blood circulation in the pelvis minor may also have a harmful influence, for example in the case of permanent sedentary work or lack of exercise.

One would not believe, but we can even have an influence on the condition of our perineal muscles with ***our clothing***. If we often wear tight underwear, tight-fitting trousers, the blood supply of our pelvic muscles will be inadequate as a result of the pressure; the oxygenation worsens resulting in the declining of muscular strength as well. Only the muscle / organ adequately supplied with blood can work properly.

The predisposing factors mentioned above refer mainly to Pelvic Floor Symptoms (urinary, bowel and sexual functions), when risk is induced by the injury or overloading of the muscles of the pelvic floor. However, Urinary Incontinence and Erectile dysfunction (ED) may also occur as a side effect of medicines.

Other reason of incontinence and ED may also be of ***neurological origin***. There are certain neurological disorders, for example sclerosis multiplex or Parkinson's disease, which are accompanied by continence and ED problems as concomitant symptom.

Having checked this list, it may be thought provoking to consider how many people are included in the at-risk group for pelvic floor dysfunction.

Why does it matter if our intimate (PC) muscles are weak?

As a result of the everyday load endured, the sphincter muscles and the supporting ligaments lose their strength. The weakening of the pelvic floor muscles may induce the following symptoms in men (even in young age):

- ***Involuntary loss of urine*** occurring with increases in intra-abdominal pressure such as a cough, laugh or strain (lifting, running, jumping);
- During urination the ***urine flow is less intense***;
- Some drops of urine leaving embarrassing ***wet urine spots on the underwear***;
- The last drops of ***urine are discharged with difficulty*** or perhaps by "shaking" only;
- ***Frequent urination*** followed by urinary incontinence;
- ***Hemorrhoids*** may develop;
- Softened testicles, ***testicle pain*** or discomfort may occur;
- Because of the weakness of the anal sphincter muscles, it may be ***difficult to control stool and gas***. The underwear may get soiled with stool in spite of proper hygiene;

- In addition to the weak pelvic floor muscles, the atonia of the connective tissue and the inadequate discharging habits, they are responsible for the development of hemorrhoids and ***varicose veins*** around the testicles. When testicular blood circulation slows down, toxins are produced in the testicles as a result of the stagnation. This causes a rise in temperature of the testicles. Accordingly, appropriate "cooling", i.e. the ideal temperature required for the production of male gametes (sperm) is not available.
- ***During erection, the angle*** formed by the penis and the abdominal wall is more obtuse than before;

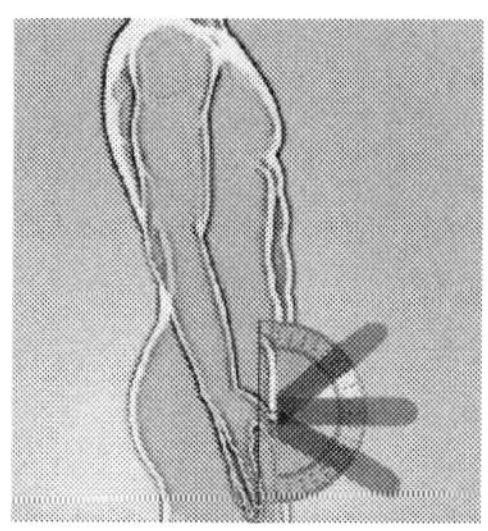

- The release of semen from the penis (***ejaculation***) during sexual intercourse or masturbation not as powerful like before, the sperm just bubbles out;
- It becomes difficult to control the erection, ejaculation and sexual activity. The hypotonicity of the blood vessels, connective tissue of the penis and the insufficient flow of blood to the penis may cause the ***inadequate hardness of the erect penis***, in spite of the libido unchanged.
- ***Several types of prostate problems*** can occur in men if the pelvic floor muscles are weak. Pelvic floor muscles work together with other pelvic organs by contracting and relaxing properly help men to urinate or defecate and during ejaculation, the prostatic fluid gets squeezed out

with the help of muscular contractions. If the pelvic floor muscles are weakened or contrariwise they are too tense or spastic, they do not work as well as they should. The accumulation and stagnation of prostatic fluid can contribute to the development of infection in the prostate. Recurrent prostatitis and Benign Prostatic Hyperplasia (BPH) are frequent diseases due to pelvic floor dysfunction.

Benign Prostatic Hyperplasia

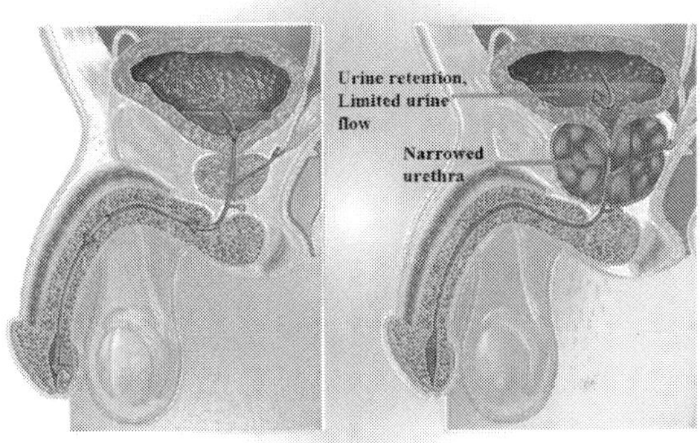

Normal Prostate Enlarged Prostate

Prostate problem can develop easily, because the prostate is an organ with a glandular substance with originally poor blood supply, since it is wedged in between the urinary bladder and the perineal muscles. Thus, the pathogenic agents can easily settle down in it. The prostatitis (inflammation of the prostate gland) is accompanied by severe perineal-, lumbar- and abdominal pain, a sense of discomfort, pain and heaviness in the area of the perineum (between the scrotum and rectum), tormenting urge to urinate, difficulty starting to urinate, stinging and burning sensation in the urethra, painful ejaculation and erection problems.

These symptoms are worth noticing! As time passes, starting with mild symptoms – in lack of abatement of the inducing factors – will mostly exacerbate. It would be a mistake to think that this is only the problem of the senior age group.

The youthfulness of the perineum is independent of age!

Perineal fitness depends only on the extent one exercises his hidden intimate muscles. The sooner you start to train the muscles of the pelvic floor, the more inconveniences you can avoid in the future.

THE UPGRADED IWT® KEGEL EXERCISES IN PRACTICE

The Teaching Methodology of IWT® (Intimate Wellness Training®) was developed from my own experiences in pelvic floor muscle training, integrated with other types of movement therapies, with the aim to strengthen the muscles of the pelvic floor in the best possible way.

IWT® first of all is a preventive method, not only trains the muscles of the pelvic floor but also part of the conscious health protection. Simultaneously with strengthening the hidden muscles of the perineum (the muscles around the root of the penis, the sphincter muscles around the anus and urethra and the muscles under the prostate), the supplementary program teaches various practices to protect the pelvic organs in order to avoid their (further) injuries.

A significant number of people with different kind of pelvic floor symptoms may feel too embarrassed to discuss their sexual, urinary and bowel issues with their healthcare providers, thinking that they have to accept their embarrassing symptoms and to live with them since they are a normal part of aging. However, it is not so!

Pelvic health is crucial for the whole body health. No matter what is our age or health history. IWT® Pelvic floor muscle training is useful not only for those who have already physical symptoms, caused by muscular weakness, but for those, who wish to preserve the strength of their perineal muscles, too.

Some tips before you start the exercise program;

- Empty your bladder before beginning the exercises.
- Turn off your mobile phone, put it into "Do Not Disturb" mode to avoid being disturbed or interrupted while you are learning the exercises.
- I advise you not to eat anything heavy 1-2 hours before the exercises. Any light meal is not causing problems.
- Be well hydrated, but please do not drink too much water before starting your workout.
- The only equipment you need is possibly an exercise mat or towel. If you have problems with your knees will be also useful to keep nearby a softer cushion.
- It is suggested to wear comfortable, loose-fitting clothing that allows you to move freely.

- Do not proceed to the next exercise section, until you are not sure doing a movement / contraction correctly.
- If you are not sure you are exercising the right muscles, put your fingertips on your perineum (between the scrotum and anal opening). You should feel a gentle squeeze under your fingertips while doing the contraction.
- After exercises, drink enough mineral water to rehydrate yourself.

Are there any contraindications?

- Opinions vary as concerns malignant (cancerous) tumors of the pelvis minor. Certain doctors would not recommend the physical training, while others claim that it may be permitted, as once a tumor is induced to grow, it will grow anyway. Knowing the fact, that the appropriate functions of the organs are ensured by the adequate circulation of blood and oxygen, I would think that physical exercise might only improve one's condition. I suggest you consult your doctor before starting the training!
- If there is a catheter introduced into the urethra, IWT® exercises are not recommended.

EXERCISES TO WARMING UP AND TO MAKE CONSCIOUS THE FUNCTION OF THE PERINEAL MUSCLES

How to develop body awareness and your ability to control the function of your muscles?

The basic requirements of learning pelvic floor exercises is to develop body awareness and your ability to control the function of your muscles, with the aim to be able to distinguish the important difference between strengthen and relaxation of muscles. So, let me present you some exercise that can help you to learn pelvic floor exercises and to feel how these little invisible perineal muscles are working.

1. Lie down in supine position (on your back) with knees bent and feet on the floor. Perform deep **abdominal breathing** 2-3 times. How to do it? Place both of your hands on your abdomen, just above your belly button. Take a slow deep breath in through your nose; you should feel your abdomen rise as your lungs fill with air; as you slowly exhale through your mouth, allow your abdominal muscles relax; your belly goes back to its normal position. It is important to let your belly to move parallel with the breath and hold the movement until a convenient time. Abdominal breathing helps to relax tense sphincter muscles.

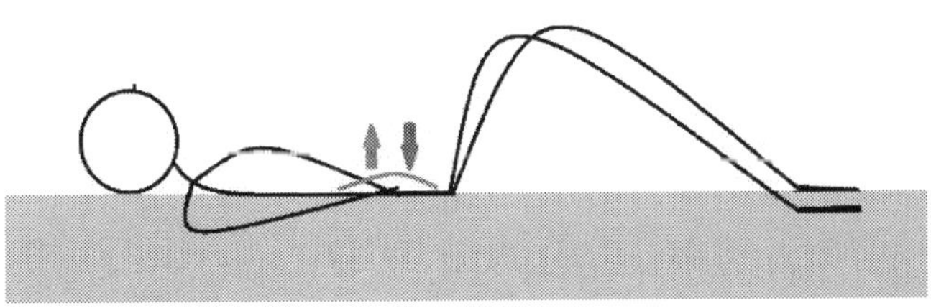

2. Remain in supine position with one leg straight and the other bent at the knee. Shoulders are relaxed, arms by the sides of the body. As you inhale, gradually raise your extended leg up to hip level by flexing back-and-forth the ankles; then, in a clockwise direction, start to rotate with your raised leg (toes are facing the ceiling) forming small circles, use the hip joint as the axis of rotation. Repeat 5- 5 times the rotation in clockwise and counter-clockwise direction. Try to keep your feet flexed. As you exhale slowly, bring your leg back to the mat. Repeat the exercise with your other leg.

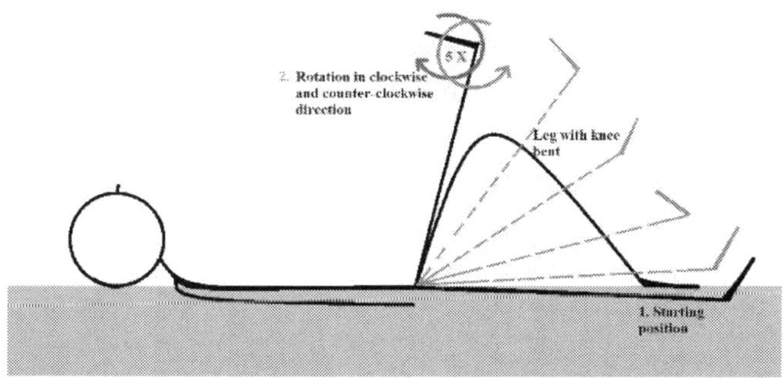

3. In supine position with knees bent, both feet flat on the mat. As you inhale, bring your right knee toward your chest, clasp your hands around the knee and pull it closer to your chest. Hold this position for a few seconds then slowly lower your right leg back to the starting position. Repeat 5 times on each leg, by alternating legs. At the end, open and close your legs 4-5 times.

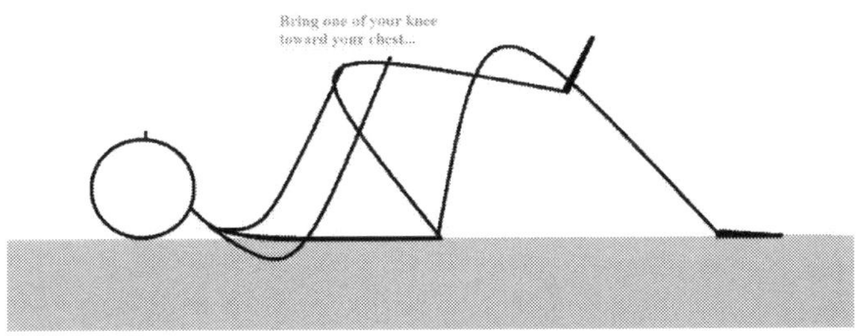

4. In the same position, slowly tighten your buttock muscles, until you feel that these muscles become harder. You can feel the gluteal muscles work if you put your hands in the middle of your buttock. Squeeze your buttocks again, you will feel the muscles go tight and hard under your hands. Relax your muscles.

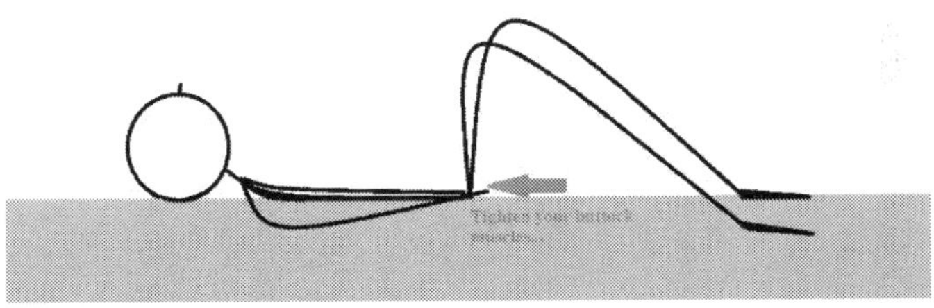

5. Place your hands on your belly, just below your navel and pay attention to your abdominal muscles. Your abdominal muscles should be soft and relaxed. Muscles should be soft when relaxed. Tightening again your buttock muscles strongly, you should feel that your lower abdominal muscles become a little bit tcnsc.

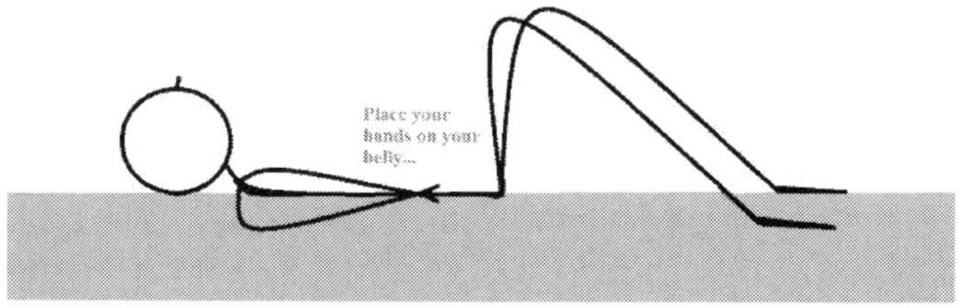

6. Raise your trunk up until your shoulder blades are off the mat. As you lift your trunk off the mat, you should feel a slight burning sensation by the lower abdominal muscles. You should feel as the lower abdominal muscles become a little bit tense. Return to the starting position and relax your muscles.

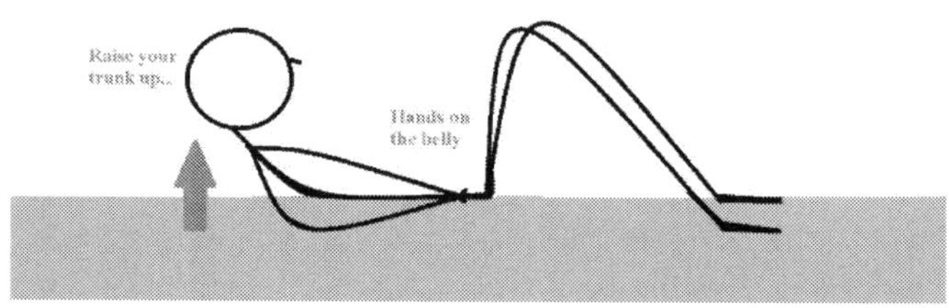

7. Remain in supine position with knees bent; imagine a wet sponge placed between your knees. Place the palms of your hands on your inner thigh muscles. Try to “dry” completely the sponge with squeezing strongly your knees and thighs together. You should feel as the inner thigh muscles become tighter and firmer. When you spread your legs in hip-distance apart, you can feel the inner thigh muscles become

relaxed and loose. Did you feel with your hand the difference between the tense state and the relaxed state of your muscles?

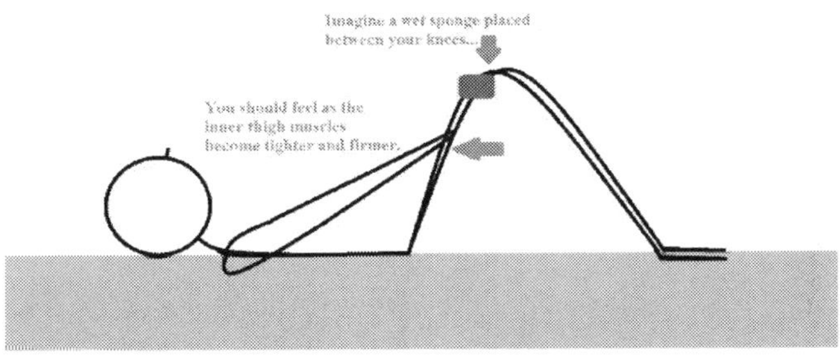

EXERCISES TO MAKE CONSCIOUS THE MOVEMENTS OF THE EXTERNAL ANAL SPHINCTER MUSCLE

To the following exercises at the beginning, it is important to work slowly with a lot of patience. First, you will learn how to perceive and voluntarily move the sphincter muscle around the anus, the muscles around the penis and under the prostate, one by one at the beginning than the whole musculature of the pelvic floor. After, you gradually get to know finer exercises aimed at more skillful and stronger motions. At first, you may find to carry out the required exercise impossible, but it will be still possible by the stepped structure of the training of the IWT® technique. Having the proper information, the exercises - initially considered difficult to carry out – can be learned quickly and safely by everyone.

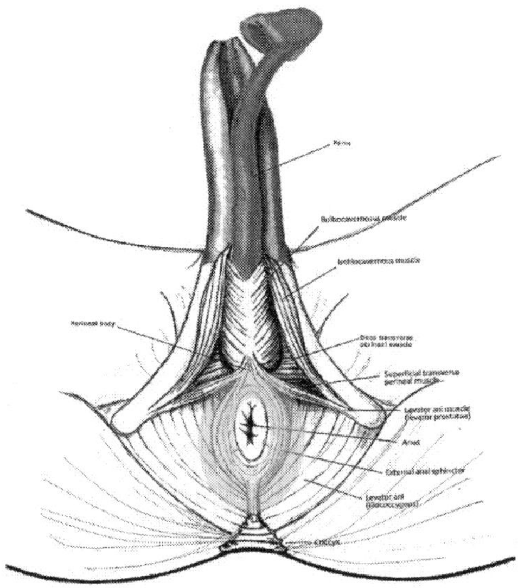

First, you should pay attention to the movements of your anal orifice. You have to learn step by step how to squeeze the muscles around the anus in the proper way.

You should observe in different postures the sensations, that you feel during the contractions of the anal sphincter muscle, afterwards you should settle yourself in that posture in which you felt better the movements of the external anal sphincter muscle.

Lie on your side with your body in a straight line, keep your bottom leg straight, the upper knee is comfortably flexed and raised toward your chest. Allow your flexed leg to slide in front of the supporting straight leg.

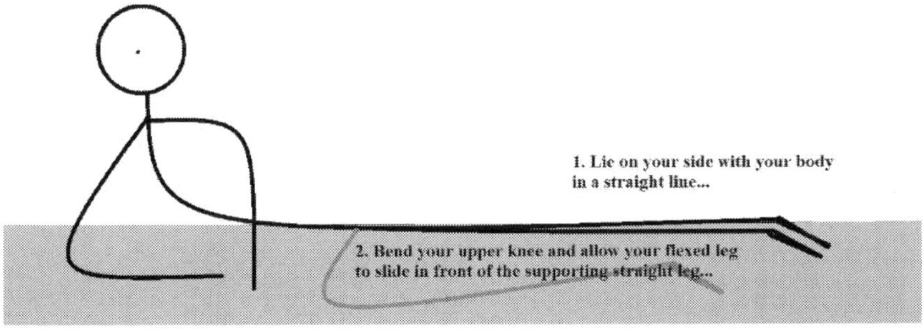

Palpation is a powerful tool for training muscles. After we have felt the contraction of a muscle, we are able to contract a muscle properly and to perceive the difference between a weak and strong contraction or between contraction and relaxation.

Place your three central fingertips over the anus *(DO NOT INSERT YOUR FINGER INTO YOUR RECTUM!), from any direction,* ***over your clothes****.*

The fingertips should only feel the contraction of the anal sphincter muscle. It is important to check the movements of the perineal muscles with your hand, just to be sure, if you actually are doing correctly the contraction of the anal sphincter muscle, because later, every other exercise will be based on this basic movement.

1. **Perform some imitating movement of stool retention. It means, try to tighten the sphincter muscle around the anus, as though you are trying to keep under control an urge of diarrhea or as if you are trying to stop passing gas (at this moment do not pay attention to the movements of the**

penis or scrotum). Pay attention only to the movement that you feel under your fingertips.

Perform this imitation movement of stool retention several times, until you are sure, you are exercising the correct muscle. Tightening the sphincter muscle of the anus should be felt at fingertips only. Try to "work" only with the perineal muscles and let the surrounding muscles like the inner thighs, belly or buttocks in relaxed state. You should feel only the intimate muscles working between your legs. Do not hold your breath while squeezing! Try to breathe normally.

Please do not be discouraged if at the beginning you do not perceive clearly the movements. Even people with very weak pelvic muscles can be taught these exercises. Maybe your pelvic muscles still are not strong enough, but their force can be developed easily if you are diligent and you will perform IWT® exercises regularly.

Correct movements:

- In case of a correct movement, parallel with the contraction of the anal sphincter, your anal opening is tightly closed, the circular sphincter muscle around your anus is retracting, moving up toward the abdominal cavity, upwards, away from your underclothes. You can feel the occlusion movement of the anal opening or its upward movement. Check out both kinds of movement with your fingertips. Pay attention to how the muscles around your anus get tighter as you squeeze them and how the anal opening moves up, away from your underwear.

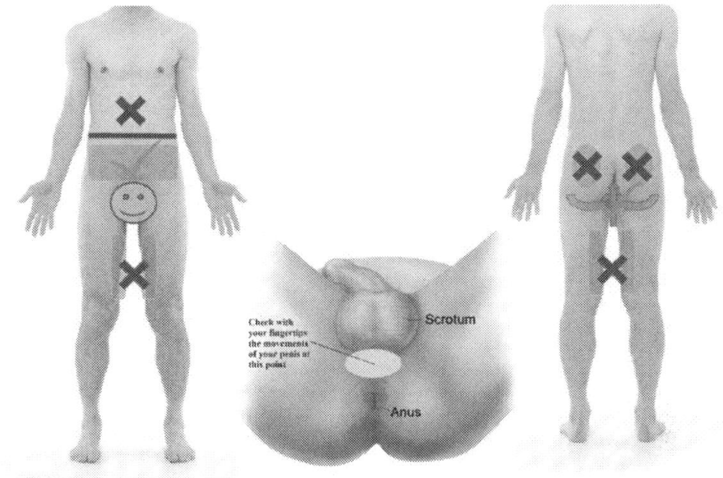

- The inner curves of your buttock participate in the movement. If you do the muscle contraction correctly, every time when you tight the muscles around the anus, the inner parts of your buttock approach to each other, but your gluteal muscles should remain relaxed as much as possible. The visible or palpable contraction of the gluteal or inner thigh muscles, which accompanies the internal pelvic floor contraction, is not incorrect, but makes the learning process or the identification of pelvic floor muscles much more difficult. To avoid the contraction of the gluteal or inner thigh muscles, at the beginning try not to tighten your pelvic muscles strongly, just until you can feel their movements.
- During the contraction of the anal sphincter muscle, the lower abdominal muscles may be tightened a bit below the belly button, in a visible or palpable way, regardless of your will. That is fine. Of course, you can also feel the movement of your penis or scrotum does not matter!

- You should perform closure or retention movement, it is very important to tighten the right muscles and to perform the squeeze properly.

Incorrect movements:

You are not doing the contraction of the anal sphincter muscle in the proper way if:

- You push down your anal sphincter muscle instead of squeezing and lifting up, therefore during the squeeze, the anal orifice is opening like during evacuation.
- You are using a forced movement to tighten the circular sphincter muscle around your anus; it may cause hemorrhoids.
- Your chest rises or moves down while you are squeezing your pelvic floor muscles.
- If you are tightening your upper abdominal muscles (above your belly button) then you are trying too hard to squeeze the pelvic muscles!
- The gluteal muscles are hardening.
- You hold back your breath while doing a contraction.

Check out the squeeze of the anal sphincter also in supine position.

Lie on your back with knees bent, feet flat on the floor. Place knees and feet hip-distance apart, arms beside your body.

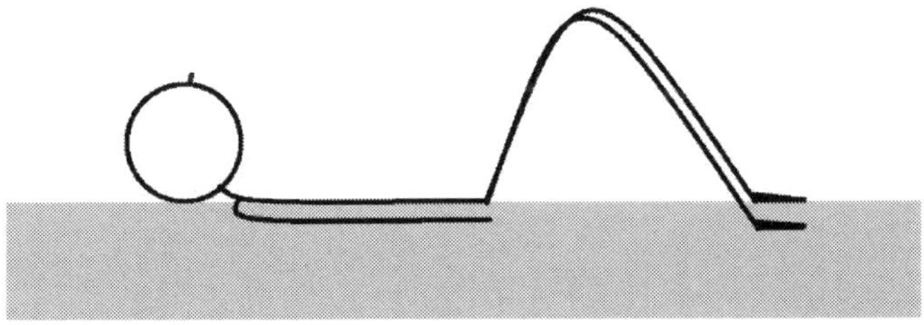

If you are sure that you are able to squeeze your anal sphincter muscle correctly, you do not need to check its movements with your fingertips anymore.

Repeat the exercise described above also in the all fours position, the thighs and arms upright, keep your back and shoulders straight.

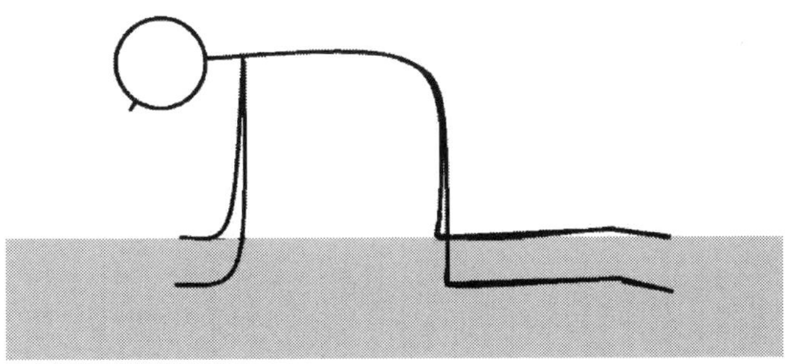

Did you feel the movements of your anal sphincter muscle?

Now settle yourself into that position, in which you have felt better the movements of the anal sphincter muscle or in which you could tighten the muscles around your anus firmly.

You can assume the supine position with knees bent, the side-lying position, or the "on all fours" position.

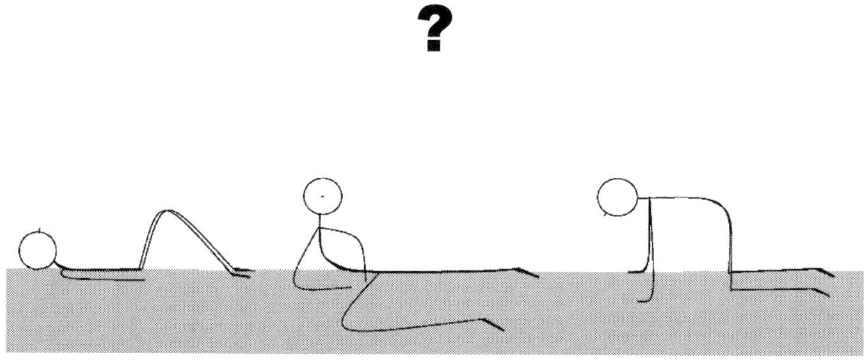

The comfortable posture is important, because if you feel uncomfortable in a posture while doing exercises, then you are unable to focus on what you are doing.

If you cannot decide, I suggest you to settle yourself in supine position with knees bent.

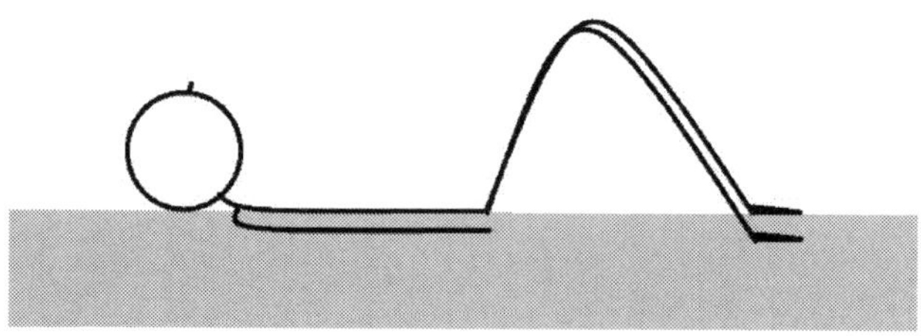

In the next step, you should squeeze the circular sphincter muscle around the anus in the same way like before, but this time try to tighten your anal sphincter muscle with your maximum force (maximum squeeze).

A muscle's ability to contraction, dependent upon its length or degree of contraction. To achieve strength and muscle development, the contraction of the muscle should be done with maximum force. It develops only that muscle fiber which is contracted, so that is why you have to try to squeeze your anal sphincter muscle, as strongly as you can. Try not to hold your breath while doing the contraction.

2. **Try to relax your abdominal muscles. Focus only on the sphincter muscle ring around your anus. Squeeze tightly the sphincter muscle around the anus, pull it up and in. Check out if you are able to increase more the strength of the contraction, lifting the sphincter muscle up more inside. Now relax your muscle ring around your anus. Slow elongated exhalation, almost like a sigh of relief. You should have a definite feeling of letting go.**

Attention! Try to apply the contraction with the maximum force only by the hidden pelvic floor muscles; you should feel the muscles working only between your legs! Pay attention to your pelvis, do not tighten your buttock or inner tight muscles or pull in your abdomen. In the beginning, use your hands to control the correct movements. Put your hands on the buttocks or inner thighs, to make sure that you are using your hidden pelvic muscles indeed!

If you have chosen another position before, to the next exercise, please settle yourself in supine position with knees bent.

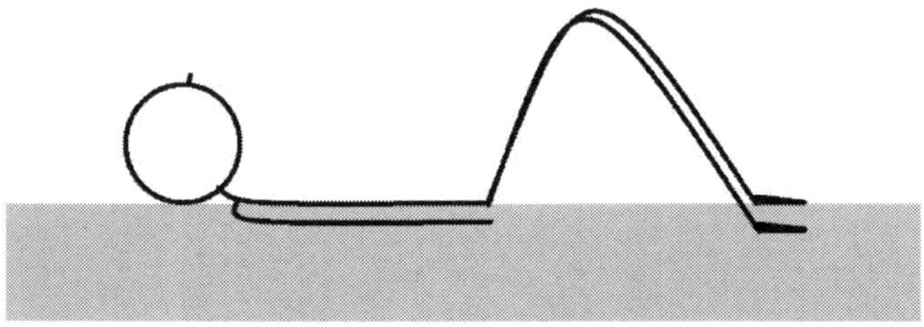

3. **You should repeat the previous exercise, with a strong contraction of the anal sphincter muscle, but this time please, pay attention consciously to that, how these pelvic muscles return back to their relaxed state after a strong contraction. You should feel during the relaxation period, how your anal sphincter muscle releasing the tension, returns to its normal relaxed state, to the direction of your underwear. You should have a definite feeling of letting go.**

Of course, you do not have to be afraid you will have an "accident" by relaxing your anal sphincter muscle. In fact, in case of evacuation, should relax also the internal anal sphincter muscle and its function is independent of our will, it will open only after the evacuation reflex.

In the intimate gymnastics, the relaxation of the pelvic floor muscles has the same importance as the quality of the contraction. In case of a muscle contraction, due to the increased pressure, the constriction of blood vessels decreases the transport of nutrients and oxygen, while the complete relaxation of the muscles allows faster blood flow, providing sufficient energy and nutrition for the active muscles and to the next contraction. Who wants to train his pelvic floor muscles tightening only without relaxing completely, the muscles will remain slightly contracted, impeding the sufficient blood flow to the muscle fibers; therefore his muscles will develop less due to poor blood circulation.

It may happen that the relaxation of the pelvic floor muscles is more difficult than to perform the contraction itself. You can feel that your muscles are not relaxed completely; you perceive as an unpleasant sense of tension. In this case, to help to relax your tense muscles, separate your knees a few times as wide as comfortable or perform some abdominal breathing. (You can find the description above by the warm up exercises)

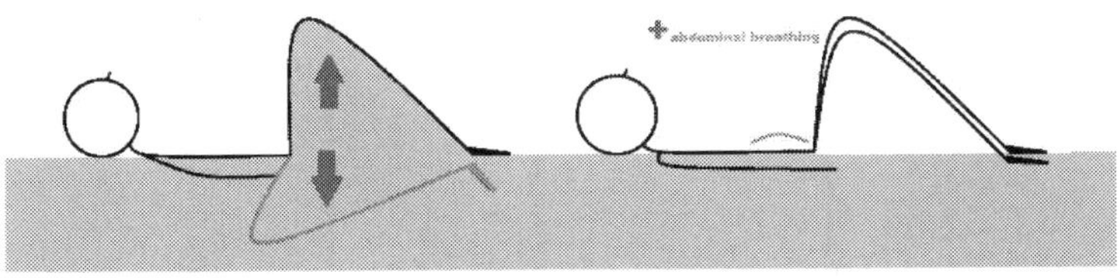

4. **Until now, you had to pay attention how your external anal sphincter muscle can be tightened and relaxed. Now you should perform the contraction of the anal sphincter muscle slowly, gradually and consciously, observing the phases of the contraction. The contraction of the anal sphincter muscle should be gradual from the relaxed state of the muscle until reaching the maximal strength of contraction without stopping at the different phases of the contraction!**

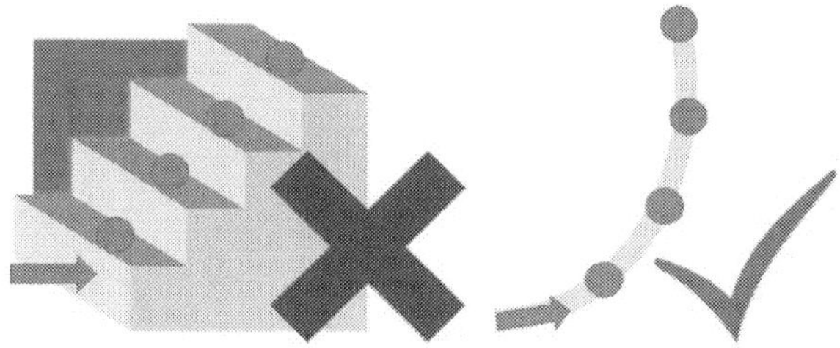

- Initially, the anal sphincter muscle is in a relaxed state,
- the anal sphincter muscle leaves the state of immobility; at this point, you should pay attention to that feeling when "the sphincter muscle just moves slightly",
- continuing the squeeze of the sphincter muscle, you arrive till the half strength of the maximal force,
- still increasing the force of the contraction of the anal sphincter muscle, you can perceive to tighten the circular muscle almost with your maximum force,
- going further with the contraction, try to get till your maximum force and then let to relax completely the muscles around your anus.

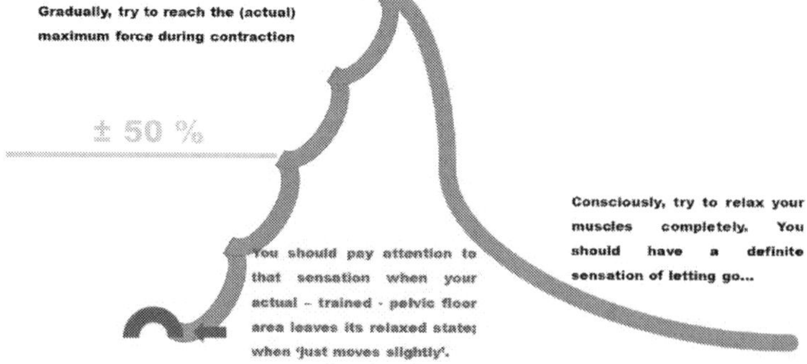

If you lose meantime the strength of the contraction, no problem, just squeeze your sphincter muscle again and continue to perform the exercise.

5. **Repeat the previous exercise, but after reaching the maximum force of contraction, performed slowly, gradually counting to 4, try to hold the most intensive contraction counting to 4, finally relax your muscles gradually counting as well to 4.**

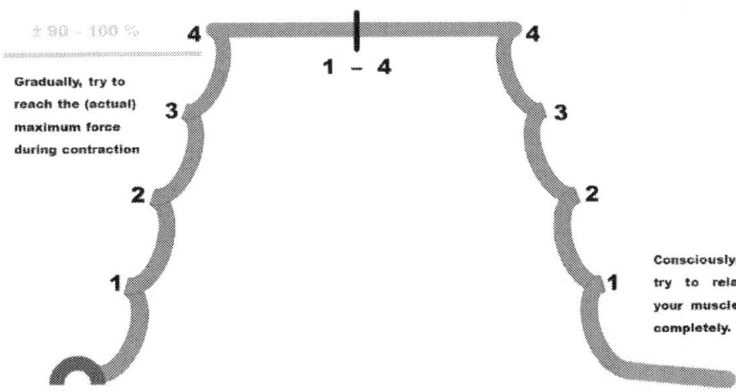

If you feel, that despite of your efforts, your sphincter muscle loosens up unintentionally, you lose the strength of the contraction, means that your perineal muscles are not enough strong yet. No problem. Squeeze your anal sphincter muscle again and continue to perform the exercise.

It could happen that at the first attempt you will not able to perform this exercise successfully. This is because of the weakness of the pelvic floor muscles. Usually the easiest thing is to manage the gradual contraction of muscle. As your pelvic muscles get stronger, it will be also easier to hold the strength of the contraction for longer time, and the ability to relax your muscles gradually and slowly will develop last.

In the next step, you should make the contraction of the anal sphincter muscle with a posterior pelvic tilt.

How to do a posterior pelvic tilt?

Let's see the movement of the pelvis. Pay careful attention to the sequence of the movement:

> **In supine position. First, breathe in, start the pelvic tilt movement as you exhale. Parallel with the exhalation slowly begin to tilt your pelvis backwards, flatten your lower back against the mat by tightening your abdominal muscles and bending your pelvis up slightly, but your buttocks should not lift off the floor. When you blow out the air, your abdomen should come toward your back automatically. In this position, you cannot put your hand under your lower back (under the curve in the lumbar spine) CHECK IT! In this position, you should not be able to place your hands under your lower back. As you exhale, allow the spine and pelvis to return to their original – neutral position.**

Posterior Pelvic Tilt

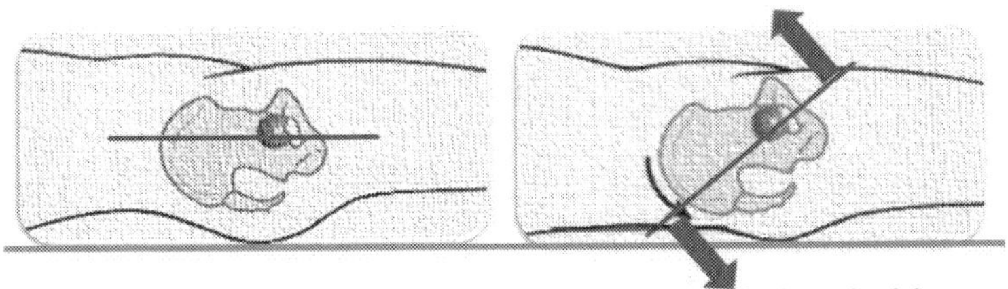

Natural curve of the lower spine

The curve of the lower back is decreased, your lower back should be flat against the floor

! Do not hold your breath while performing the pelvic tilt.

Perform this pelvic tilt a few times or until you feel confident with the movement. Even though the movement is simple, it can prove very difficult to do in practice. Be patient with yourself.

To make more powerful the contraction of the pelvic floor muscles you should learn also **the posterior pelvic tilt plus.**

In supine position with knees bent, feet on the floor. Begin to squeeze slightly your gluteal muscles together. At the same time, gradually start to tilt your pelvis backwards, press your lower back into the mat. In this position, the curve in your lumbar spine should straighten, and your lower back should be flat against the mat. CHECK OUT your position by trying to place your hand underneath your lower back! In this position, you should not be able to do that. Continue to tighten your buttocks till the maximum force; consequently, your belly retracts toward your spine. You should feel a stronger, deeper contraction. As you exhale, relax your

muscles and allow the spine and pelvis to return to their original – neutral position.

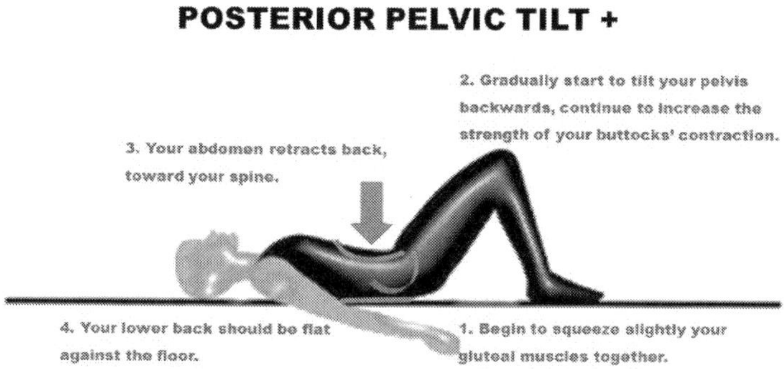

Repeat the pelvic tilt a few times or until you feel confident with the movement. Do not forget to breathe!

The purpose of the next exercise with the pelvic tilt + is, to strengthen the anal sphincter muscle more intensively, therefore you should integrate the contraction of the anal sphincter muscle with the contraction of the buttock muscles. (I asked you before, not to use your buttocks. I did it, because first you had to learn to perceive and move voluntarily your anal sphincter muscle separately.)

Let's join the pelvic tilt + with the contraction of the anal sphincter muscle!

6. **Relax your abdominal muscles. Pay attention only to the movement of your anal sphincter muscle. Tighten the muscles around your anus just slightly, hold this slight tension, squeeze your buttock muscles slightly together – simultaneously move your pelvis backward and press the lower back down into the mat, increase**

the force of contraction of your buttock till the maximum force, squeeze your anus muscles as strongly as you can, lift them up and inside as high as you can, check if you can squeeze it even more. As you exhale relax your muscles. Let your abdominal muscles become soft, slow elongated exhalation, almost like a sigh of relief. Allow the spine and pelvis to return to their original – neutral position.

Keep in mind! Even during a maximal squeeze, you should work only with your pelvic floor muscles!

7. **Repeat the previous task with a pelvic tilt +, but trying to keep the maximal contraction for a count of 4.**

8. **Now, perform 8 definite, short, fast and strong contractions with your anal sphincter muscle, as quickly as you can. Do not try to hold on to the contractions; just squeeze and relax. Remain in supine position, with knees bent. In order to maintain a balance, place your arms on the floor alongside your body, palms facing down. As you exhale press your feet into the floor, slowly lift your pelvis up off the mat into a bridge, your pelvis is in line with your shoulders and knees, hold this position for 10 seconds. Remember to breathe! Release and roll slowly back down to the**

floor. Inhale deeply through your nose into your abdomen and slowly blow out the air while you relax your pelvis completely, this deep abdominal breath relaxes the muscles that are not under your conscious control.

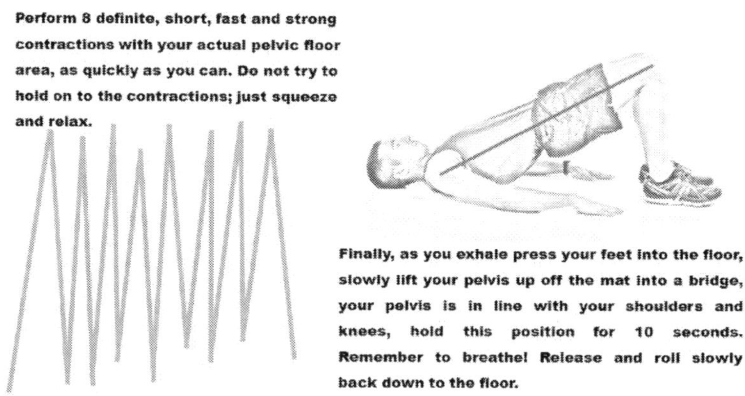

**If you cannot hold this position, as an alternative you can place a cushion under your buttocks to keep them raised*

EXERCISES TO MAKE CONSCIOUS THE MOVEMENTS OF THE MUSCLES AROUND THE PENIS AND UNDER THE PROSTATE GLAND

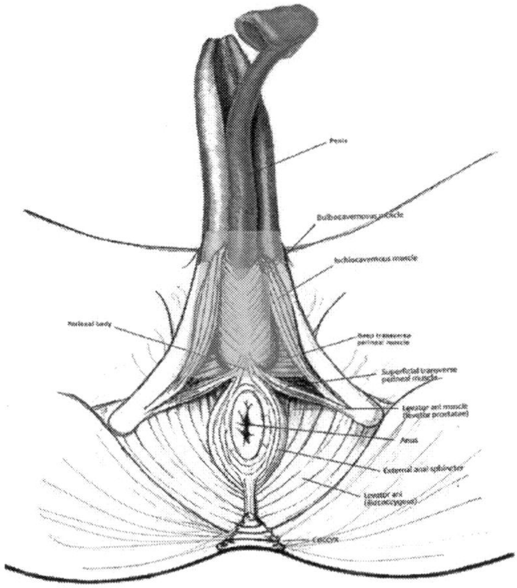

It may seem an unusual idea that one should care about the training of the muscles around the penis and rectum or those below the prostate, but this is a primary condition of the proper function of these parts of the body even in elderly age. The erection height of the penis could be preservable throughout the whole life, if the muscles around the penis were strong enough. In lack of training, because of the weakening of the lateral muscles, the erection angle changes in time. If the blood circulation of the penis is not satisfactory, that may often have a negative influence on sexual vigour, too.

Now, you should to pay attention only to the movements of your penis. The task will be the following: meanwhile you will tighten rhythmically your anal sphincter muscle, you should pay attention to, how the muscles around and in your penis relax and contract parallel too.

Position yourself on knee-elbow position. Keep your legs and knees in hip distance apart, to be able to palpate the muscles at the base of your penis. Place your three middle fingertips at the base of your penis, close to the scrotum, over your clothes. Stay in this position.

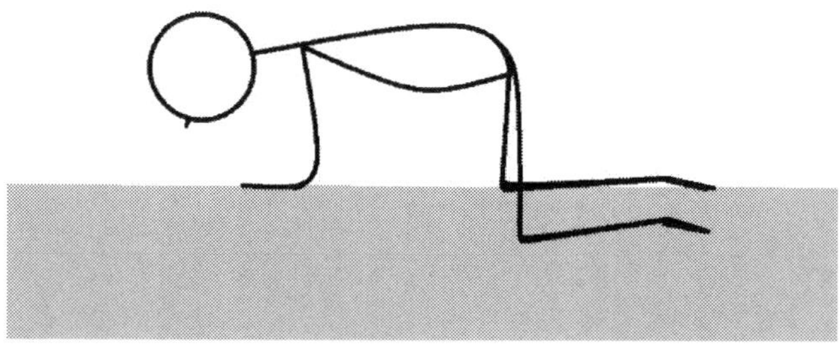

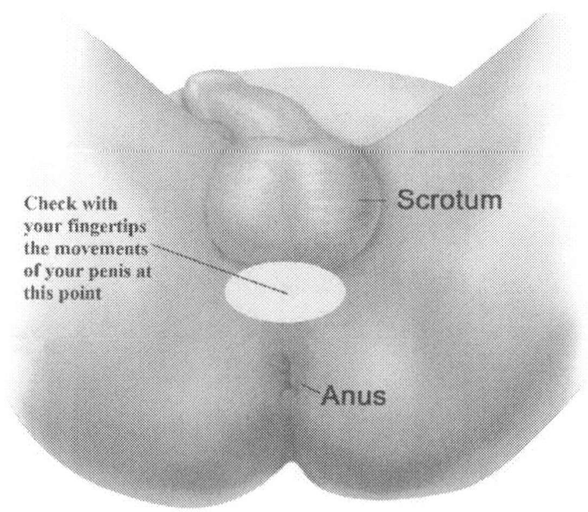

1. **Relax your abdominal muscles. Begin to squeeze your anal sphincter muscle rhythmically, like fast eye blinking. Quickly and repeatedly, squeeze the muscles around your anus. In the meantime, pay**

attention to what you perceive under your fingertips. After a few contraction, hold the squeeze of your anal sphincter muscle for a moment and meantime you relax it; try to pay attention to how the muscles around and in your penis become also relaxed. What do you feel around and in your penis when you relax the muscles around your anus?

! Do not tighten your buttock or inner tight muscles or pull in your abdomen!

Next step. In the same position, you should imitate that muscle movement, when you stop the urine flow. It may be confusing that meantime you are trying to pay attention to the movements of the urethra and penis your anal sphincter muscle is going to move, but try not to devote any attention to its movement.

2. **Relax your abdominal muscles. To move the base of your penis, start to imitate that contraction when you consciously want to stop the urine flow. Imagine that someone walks into your bathroom while you are urinating (peeing) and you need to stop your urine flow, then restarting it. Squeeze rhythmically those muscles that you would use if you were trying to hold back urine. If your technique is correct, each time when you tighten your pelvic floor muscles you may feel that the base of your penis move up slightly towards your abdomen. Pay attention to the movements that you feel under your fingertips. After a few contraction, hold the squeeze of the urethra for a moment and as you relax it, pay attention to how the muscles relax around and in your penis. You**

should feel a pleasant sensation of relaxation in your penis. When you relax the muscles around and in your penis you should feel a sensation of 'letting go'.

! You can do this urine stop test "for real" if you wish, but try to do it only ONCE, just to feel which muscles are the correct ones to use. Do not do this regularly because you may start retaining urine or it may interfere with normal bladder emptying. Once you have found the right muscles, make sure you relax and empty your bladder completely.

Correct movements:

- Imagine the muscles around your penis. When you contract these muscles, it gives a similar sensation that you feel when actually you squeeze the base of the penis with your hand.
- In parallel with the contraction of your anal sphincter muscle, also the muscles around your penis will be squeezed. You can feel that, meantime your anus continues to tighten up and relax the muscles around and in your penis are moving with the same rhythm. The sensation of warm that generated during the activity of the pelvic floor muscles provides support to the perception of the correct muscles to use.
- You may feel that your penis "pull in" slightly and your scrotum lifts up slightly, or your penis will twitch and contract in towards your body, the muscles at the base of the penis get tighter, moves slightly backward towards the rectum with each contraction of the anus.

- If you are standing in front of the mirror (with no clothes on) and tighten the right muscles, you should see the base of the penis draw in and scrotum lift up a little bit.

Incorrect movements:

- If simultaneously with the movement of the penis you feel that your anal orifice opens, like to evacuate or moves down.
- It is a mistake to pull your belly in, because in this case also the muscles around your penis will tense up.

Now, please lie on your back with knees bent. Make sure you feel comfortable.

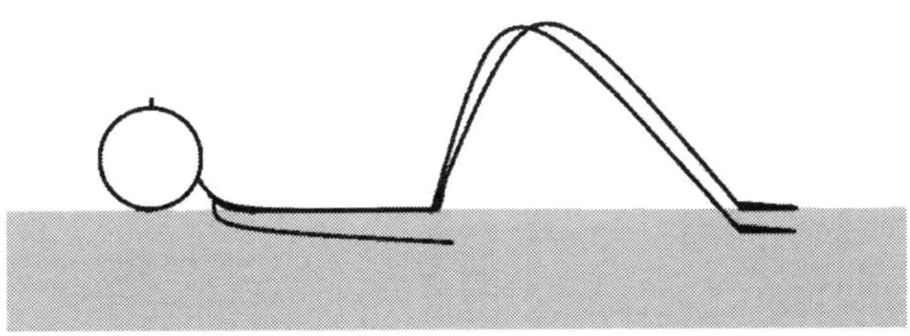

You just have observed separately the movements of the anal sphincter and the muscles around the penis. In this exercise, you should observe how these two muscle areas are moving together. This area is similar to two circles, which represent the number 8. The point where these two muscle areas are connected can be found just below the prostate gland. This is the deepest part of the pelvic floor, where connects the muscles around the penis, anus and the muscles below the prostate.

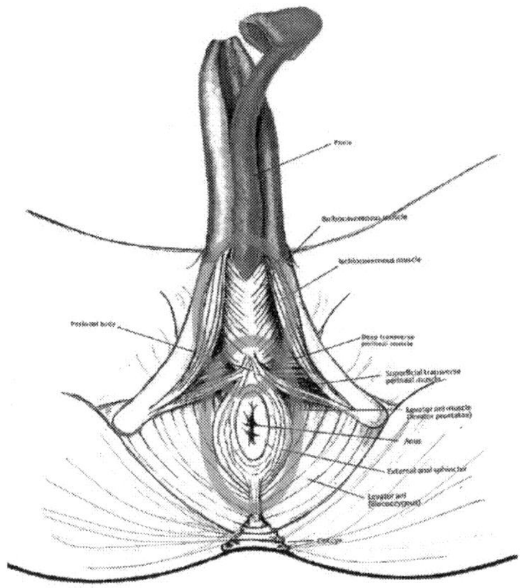

The pelvic floor is a contiguous area of muscles, like an elastic rubber band or a kind of hammock, if you begin to move on one side of this muscle area it is going to function also on the other side. When you raise up the two end points of the pelvic floor area then also its center point will be raised up.

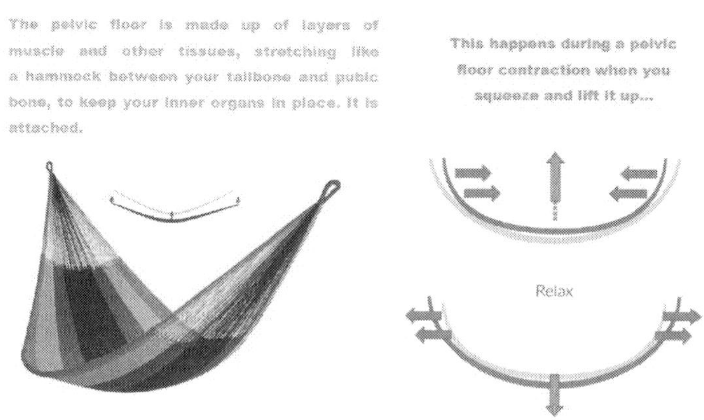

If you raise up with a contraction in front the “circle” that surrounds the penis and the “circle” behind that surrounds the anus, then you will also raise up the central point between these two end points.

You can perform the contraction squeezing both muscle areas simultaneously or first you can check the contraction of one muscle area and only after to squeeze the other muscle area. Both are appropriate solutions.

Try to “surround” both of circle’s movement with your attention. Try to imagine the muscles around the penis and the muscles around the anus.

3. **Relax your abdominal muscles. You should perform a contraction with medium force that imitates that movement when you consciously want to stop the urine flow and try to perform simultaneously the other squeeze that imitates the movement when you want to stop passing gas or hold a bowel movement until you reach a toilet. You should feel that you are squeezing both muscle “circles”. If you are sure that you have contracted both areas, relax your pelvic floor muscles.**

4. **Repeat the previous task, but this time, observe consciously how the “point” below the prostate gland is raising and how descends back to its normal position.**

Now, you should tighten the muscles around your penis with your maximum force. It is required to squeeze every single muscle around the penis that is capable of functioning, so you should look up your limits to which point you are able to squeeze the muscles around your penis.

When you squeeze the muscles around the penis, it is very important to observe every possible movement and to find the point where you can still strengthen on the squeeze, for example; if you still can lift a little bit more up the scrotum or if you still can pull back more the base of the penis toward the rectum. Of course, these are not very conspicuous movements; you do not have to be afraid from that your penis is going to move from its "normal place". These are only small checkpoints, trying to make more effective the quality of the contraction.

How to squeeze correctly the muscles around the penis with maximum force?

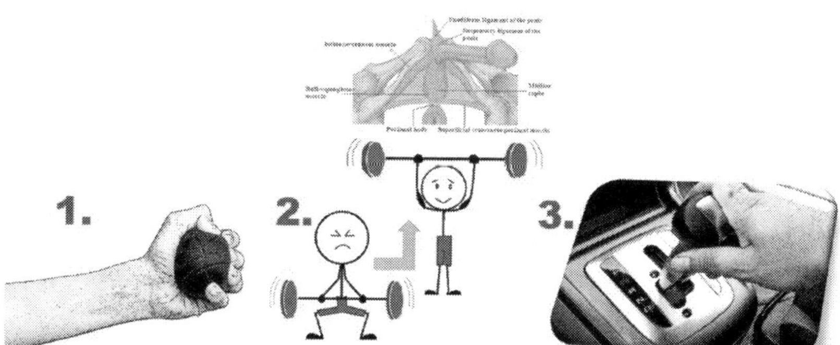

Squeeze gently the muscles around the penis, as though you are trying to stop the flow of urine.

Try to increase the force of the contraction and to 'lift' the scrotum up, as 'high' as you can.

Try to strengthen the contraction a little bit more and to 'pull' the base of the penis back, toward the rectum, just like when you change gears.

I have previously mentioned, that a muscle fiber develops only is it is fully contracted. Using a less intensive muscle contraction, the weak part of the muscle remains passive, which means that exactly the weak part of the muscle will not be able to improve in its strength.

5. **Relax your abdominal muscles. Focus only on the muscles around the penis. Begin to squeeze repeatedly the muscles around your penis, as though you are trying to stop the flow of urine. Do not try to squeeze too hard, just with moderate force. Pay attention to, how the muscles around and in your penis are contracted. You can perceive a kind of circular tight, as if the muscles around the penis would restrict in circular form or you may have a sensation as if the base of the penis would be squeezed, it is like squeezing toothpaste from a tube. If you feel the squeeze - closure at the base of your penis, or you feel a scrotal lift, hold the contraction for a moment, and just like when you pull the gear stick back in a car ("old school"), try to pull back with all your force the base of your penis, toward the rectum, try to lift up more the scrotum. Now relax the muscles around your penis, let your abdominal muscles become soft. Slow elongated exhalation, almost like a sigh of relief. You should have a definite feeling of letting go.**

! Try to avoid holding your breath, tighten your buttocks, squeeze your legs together or pulling in your abdomen. You should work only with your internal pelvic muscles.

6. **Repeat the previous exercise, but at this time follow consciously with your attention the relaxation of the muscles around and in your penis and under the prostate. Pay attention to the pleasant sensation of relaxation as your muscles spread, how the sense of the tension in your penis**

disappears completely and the scrotum descends back to its place.

If you want to be sure that your urethra should be relaxed then let your belly to relax. You may have already noticed that, when you squeeze the pelvic floor muscles, also your lower abdominal muscles become tense a bit unintentionally. The lower abdominal muscles are moving, activating together with the pelvic floor muscles even when they relax. The feeling of the relaxation of the urethra is similar to that pleasant feeling that accompanies urination.

! Do not use your buttock or inner thigh muscles! It is a mistake to pull your abdomen in, because in that case also the muscles surrounding your penis will tense up.

7. **Now you should squeeze the muscles around your penis with awareness; slowly and gradually up till your maximum force counting to 4, after try to hold your strongest squeeze counting as well to 4, and at the end slowly and gradually relax the muscles around and in your penis counting to 4. As you relax your penis muscles, pay attention to perform a prolonged exhalation, almost like a sigh. The slow and prolonged exhalation helps to turn on our parasympathetic nervous system- thereby also helps to relax body muscles.**

! Always relax your abdominal muscles before tightening the pelvic floor muscles.

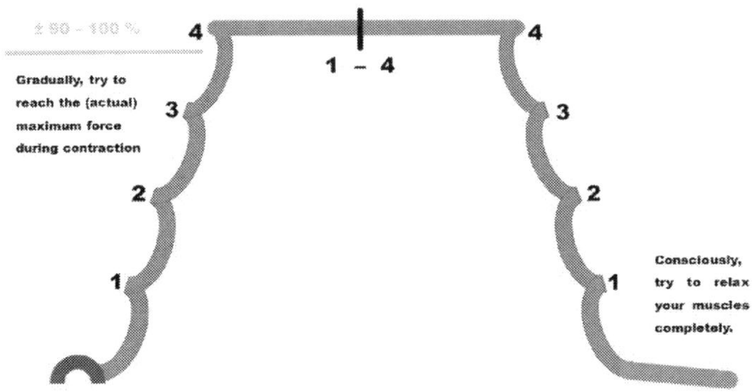

In the following exercise, you should apply an anterior pelvic tilt.

How to do an anterior pelvic tilt?

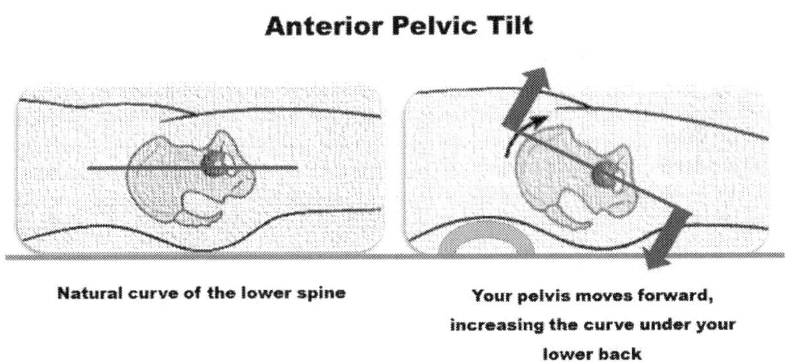

Anterior movement of the pelvis means, that your pelvis moves forward, increasing the curve under your lower back.

In standing position, if the abdomen protrudes forward contributing to an imbalance in the muscles in the pelvis and hip area. Excessive anterior pelvic tilt can contribute greatly to postural dysfunction like, lower back pain, knee pain, flat feet, hip pain, pelvic organ prolapse etc. In this exercise, the anterior pelvic tilt in supine position will be applied for therapeutic purpose.

Let's see the exercise with the movement of the pelvis. Pay careful attention to the sequence of the movements:

8. **In supine position with knees bent, feet flat on the floor. Relax your abdominal muscles. Pay attention only to the muscles around your penis. Squeeze the muscles around and in your penis just a little bit, hold this slight tension. Move your pelvis forward, in this position there is a small "bridge" under the lower back - Check out with your hand! You should not have a problem to insert your hand under your lower spine. – Stay in this position. – Increase the force of the contraction of the muscles around your penis till the maximum force; squeeze your penis tightly, "lift" the scrotum up as high as you can, "pull back" the base of your penis toward the rectum. Hold the strongest squeeze counting to 4, try to squeeze your penis in its full-length. As you exhale, slowly gradually relax your penis muscles, let your abdominal muscles become soft, slow elongated exhalation. Allow the spine and pelvis to return to their original – neutral position.**

! Do not hold your breath while performing the pelvic tilt.

Perform this pelvic tilt a few times or until you feel confident with the movement.

ANTERIOR PELVIC TILT

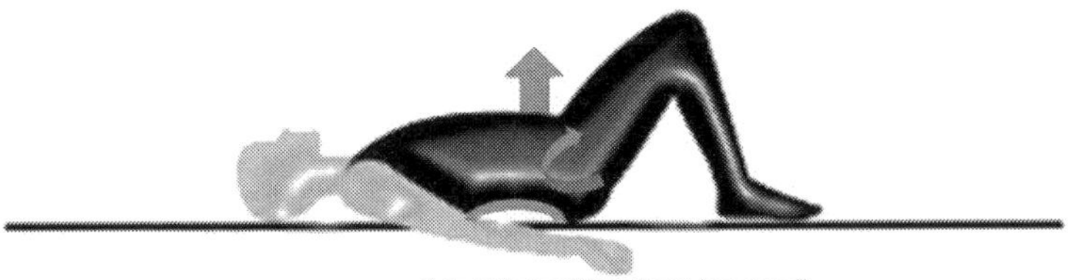

The next exercise has a very beneficial effect to support the health of the prostate gland and testicles. With the movement, generated in front of and behind your prostate, you can massage easily the prostate internally, helping to improve its blood flow, along with relieving the symptoms of prostatitis and muscular tension.

Before you have observed how the anal sphincter muscle and the muscles around the base of your penis are working with different intensity. In this exercise, you should perform one small squeeze with the muscles around and in your penis and one with your anal sphincter muscle alternately, one after the other.

9. **In supine position with knees bent. Once you "lift up" the anterior muscle area, then the posterior one. Repeat this movement a few times.**

You may feel that the muscles under the prostate gland are not tightened with the same strength. You should only pay attention to the sensation that once are tightened with more intensity the muscles around and in your penis and other time the muscles around the anal opening, as if your perineum would swing gently, rocking back and forth.

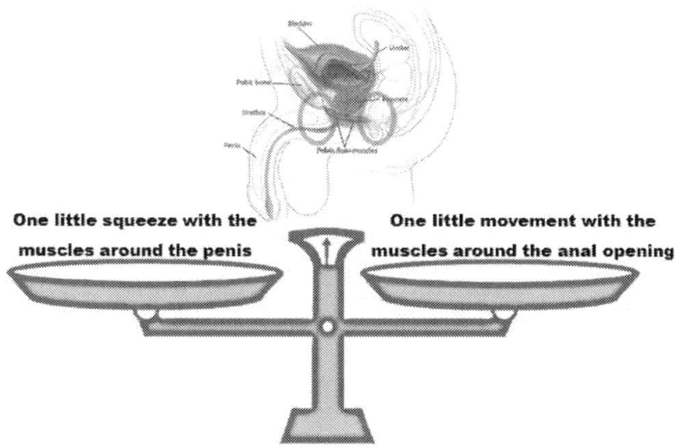

Now, hold the small squeeze in your penis counting to 4. Pay attention to the anterior part of the prostate and meantime you relax the muscles around your penis, you should pay attention where you feel a pleasant sensation. Now focus on the muscles around the anus. Squeeze the anal opening slightly, hold the tension of the anal sphincter muscle counting to 4, pay attention only to the posterior side of the prostate and relax the muscles around your anus, pay attention where you feel a pleasant sensation.

Some person, prefer to perform this exercise doing fast contractions; others prefer to do slow contractions. The rhythm in the learning phase does not matter. You should only pay attention to what you feel during the contractions. Of course, all the perineal muscles are moving together during the exercise, but the emphasis is on the direction of the movements and on the different intensity of PC-muscle squeeze. This exercise will become a strengthening exercise, when it will be performed with maximum force, but you should not do this exercise with maximum force, until you are not well trained and you do not have practice by adopting a moderate or small squeeze. If you initially, without having practice, would start to squeeze your pelvic muscles applying too much force, pelvic muscles could get strained. That is why in the learning phase you should apply only small or moderate contractions and when you will be sure, you are exercising the right muscles, you can increase the force of the contraction.

The unfavorable position of the prostate gland

The prostate has a very unfavorable position. It is located between two “waste material stores”. It is, on the one hand, pressed in between the urinary bladder and the pelvic floor muscles, forced to bear the weight of the urine contained in the urinary bladder all the time, on the other hand it is in direct connection with the rectum where our “waste products” are stored. Further, the urethra passes through the prostate and in addition to that, it should endure the continuous pressure from underneath caused by much sitting work, as well as from up, because of the wrong sitting position with curved spine which is increasing the intra-abdominal pressure.

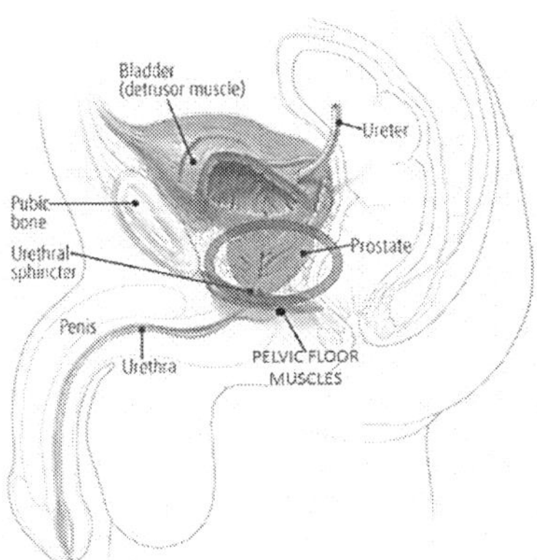

No wonder that the circulation of the prostate is always stagnant, the bacteria causing inflammation can easily settle in it, hindering its purification, prostatitis may form inside it and antibiotics can hardly reach the inner part of the prostate gland to exert their effect on it. Penile erection problems are very frequent among men doing regular sitting work, which is often accompanied by chronic prostatitis, too. Stress will only worsen the situation, since under the influence of stress the pelvic floor muscles get even tighter, hindering normal blood circulation thereby.

It is worth knowing that the greatest enemy of the prostate inflammations is to do pelvic floor exercises! If the blood circulation of the pelvic region is more vivid, the pathogenic agents will be unable to proliferate so quickly, and the tightened, tense pelvic floor muscles will relax, too. All kinds of prostate disorders caused by circulatory insufficiency can be prevented with pelvic floor exercises especially developed for men. The more intensive the squeeze of the pelvic floor muscles, the better the effect.

If you are suffering from prostatitis, you may feel the following exercise uncomfortable or unpleasant. Pain may occur, which is natural, but will cease very soon. In case of prostatitis, to avoid unbearable pains, do the following exercise with moderate intensity only.

IWT® – Flipper exercise – to massage your prostate internally

The next is a very cheerful exercise, named Flipper, with which you can massage internally your prostate very well and to improve its blood circulation. The purpose of this exercise is to move all the three muscle areas of the pelvic floor at the same time but with different intensities. This exercise has specially a strengthening effect on the central part of the perineum, the area between the anus and the scrotum, this point is called in the Far Eastern literature, "The Million Dollar Point". This point is located exactly below the prostate, pressing this point during sexual intercourse session, may help to delay ejaculation as long as you want. The prostate is sometimes referred to as the "male G-Spot". You will also be also able to delay ejaculation by tightening correctly your trained and strengthened pelvic floor muscles! You will be able to control your ejaculation more efficiently, when your pelvic floor muscles will be stronger.

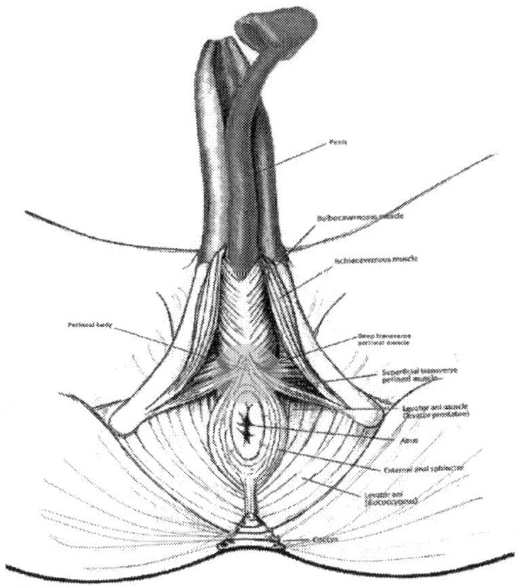

Try to imagine the three muscle areas of the pelvic floor, the muscles around and in the penis, below the prostate gland and the sphincter muscle ring around the anus.

10. Relax your abdominal muscles. Now pay attention only to the muscles around and in your penis. Try to squeeze the muscles around your penis you are your maximum force, as if you were trying to stop the flow of urine, hold the squeeze in your penis

counting to 4 and without leaving to relax the penis muscles completely, perform quickly 3 short and fast contraction with the anal sphincter muscle. Do not try to hold the contractions, just squeeze and relax.

Let's change direction.

Relax your abdominal muscles. Pay attention only to the muscle ring around your anus. Try to squeeze the muscles around your anus with maximum force, as if you're trying to hold back a bowel movement, hold the squeeze in your anus (but not buttocks!) counting to 4 and without leaving to relax your anal sphincter muscle completely, perform quickly 3 short and fast squeeze with the muscles around and in your penis. Do not try to hold the contractions, just squeeze and relax. After that, let your pelvic muscles to relax completely. As you relax your pelvic floor muscles, pay attention to perform a prolonged exhalation, almost like a sigh.

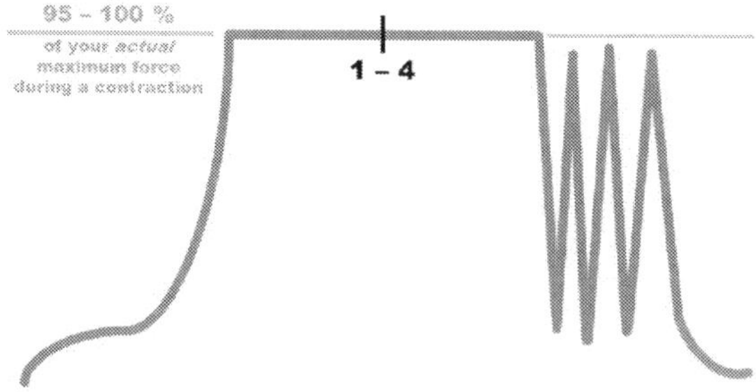

11. **Now, perform 8 definite, short, fast and strong squeeze with the muscles around the base of your penis, as quickly as you can. Do not try to hold on**

to the contractions, just squeeze and relax. Remain in supine position, with knees bent, feet flat on the floor. In order to maintain a balance, place your arms on the floor alongside your body, palms facing down. As you exhale press your feet into the floor, slowly lift your pelvis up off the mat into a bridge, your pelvis is in line with your shoulders and knees, hold this position for 10 seconds. Remember to breathe! Release and roll slowly back down to the floor. Inhale deeply through your nose into your abdomen and slowly blow out the air while you relax your pelvis completely, this deep abdominal breath relaxes the muscles that are not under your conscious control.

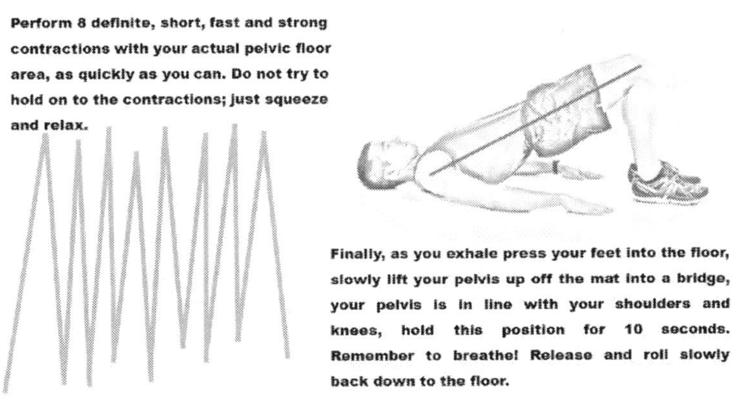

The male perineum is much more protected than the female one, which is more open and vulnerable, since it is arranged for childbirth.

The vulnerability of male organs is of a different character: the prostate is an organ with quite a poor blood supply (because of its position, sedentary lifestyle, overweight constipation etc.), which can easily get inflamed or as a result of increased loading, varicose veins may form in the region of the testicles and the rectum.

SELF- EXAMINATION

The self-examination of the testicles is inevitable. It is just as important as that of the breast or the vaginal self-examination among women. The abnormalities of the testicles can be noticed very early, making their treatment possible in due course, thus avoiding late recognition of the tumors at an advanced stage, or even the removal of one or both testicles (Orchiectomy). This self-examination might also be useful to identify other potential problems. Men periodically should check their perineal zone – at least once a month - mainly during or after a hot bath or a shower - when the scrotum relaxes and the testicles become more “visible” and palpable.

The testicles are part of the male reproductive system. This egg-shaped paired organ is the “conductor” of masculinity. It can be found in a layered tunica named scrotum. The scrotum is divided into two parts by a septum, providing separate capsules for both testicles. There are two main functions of the testicles: spermatogenesis and production of male hormone. It is the testosterone that is essentially responsible for the development and preservation of the male sex character, the masculine build, the muscular mass, muscular strength and bone mass characteristic of men and the libido, too. The lack of testosterone has a negative impact on each of these qualities and processes.

How to perform the self-examination of the testicles?

The aim of testicular self-examination is to find any suspicious nodes that might form in the scrotum. Suspicious nodes should be distinguished from epididymis, which is attached to the backside of the testis and can be touched through the skin of the scrotum.

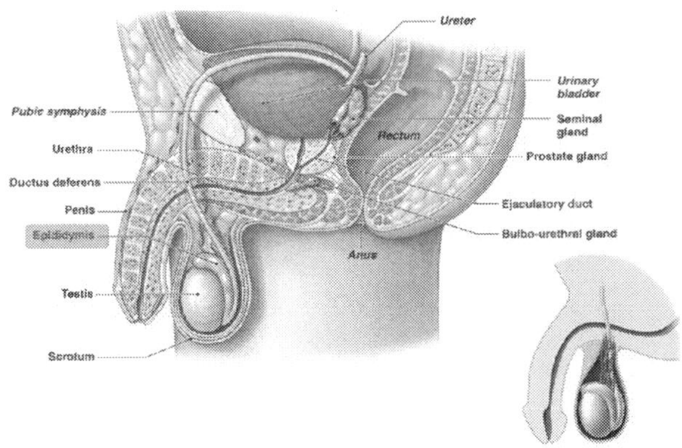

1. It is advisable to take a warm shower or bath first, as heat relaxes the scrotum and makes the examination easier.
2. If you stand in front of a mirror, you may notice any possible nodes on the scrotum more easily.
3. Gently place the testicles on your palm to feel their weight first together, then one by one. You should find if any difference or abnormality can be observed. Do not get frightened if either is bigger than the other; that is normal, but if one grows or changes in size, then that might be a warning sign.

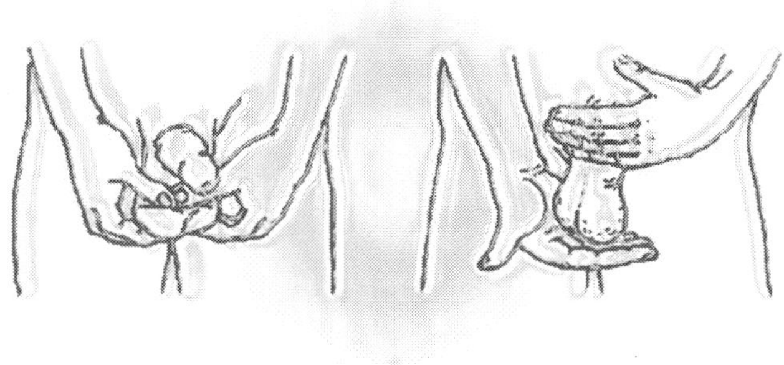

4. Both testicles should be examined separately, with two hands is possible. With great care, with fine and gentle movements touch and feel both testicles with the help of your thumb and forefinger. This way any swelling or node can be easily felt. If you come across a flexible swelling, you should not think of a tumor right away, it will prove to be hydrocele or varicocele in most cases, which can be easily removed medically. Place your forefinger and middle finger under, while your thumb on top of the testicle. This way you can gently move the testicle, feeling its smooth surface with your thumb. Your thumb will easily find the epididymis or the spermatic duct that can be found on the top of all testicles. It is easy to feel its well separable form. It should not be mixed up with any abnormal outgrowth.

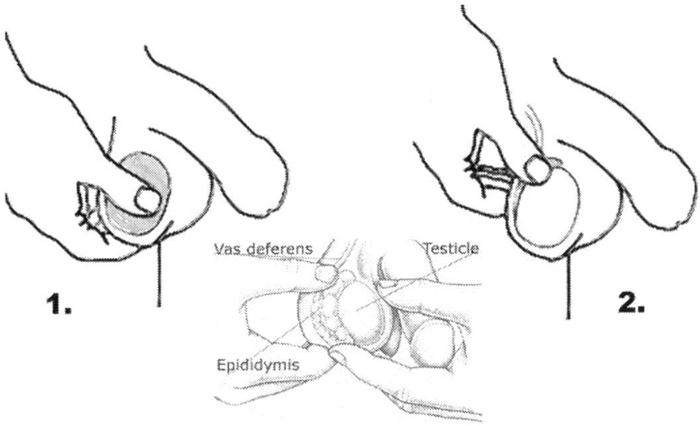

1; The surface of the testicle should be flexible and smooth. 2; The epididymis or the spermatic duct should be well separable.

5. Suspicious nodes or bumps (protuberances) can generally be found on the side of the testicle. These may be tiny (pea-size) or much larger. If you find any abnormality, consult with an andrologist or an urologist.

Varicocele is the dilatation of the testicular veins. Smaller dilatation still cannot be noticed or felt at all. Bigger ones, however, may cause serious complaints and pains. A major symptom of the disease is that after longer standing or some kind of strain, or after lifting a little heavier object; fascicular venous dilatations can be palpated or sometimes even seen over the left testicle, under the skin of the scrotum. After prolonged standing, dull slight pain may often occur in the left testicle. The significance of the varicosity of the testicular tube is that dilated veins cause worsening of the testicular blood circulation, causing a rise in temperature of the tissues surrounding the testicles. This may lead to the deterioration of spermatogenesis and testicular damage in the end. This is one of the most frequent causes of the slight deterioration of male procreativity in general. In most cases, surgery cannot be avoided even if the deviation is slight. Procreativity will be normally improving and restored after the surgery.

In most cases, when a man is operated for varicose vein of the testicle, the disease may recur in most cases in 1 or 2 years time, because he lives with similar everyday habits as before, continuing the same unhealthy routines that will end in the same problem.

! PLEASE NOTE! Under no circumstances can self-examination replace an examination by a specialist!

How to check the condition of the anal sphincter muscle?

When examining the testicles, it is advisable to check the condition of the anus, too.

Touching with a fingertip the external sphincter muscle of the anus feels hard, closing strongly even without squeezing. If you squeeze the anal sphincter muscle, it should feel closing much tighter - to a significant degree. You can have a look at it with the help of a mirror to check if you can see any bulge or protuberance around the anus. Is the region of the anal opening tender on pressure or touch? Does any bleeding occur in the rectum during defecation or the subsequent cleansing? If bleeding occurs in the anal region, you should inevitably consult a doctor, as the cause of the bleeding may only be found by proctoscopy.

When the anal sphincter loses its strength, the initial problem will be with holding the intestinal gas back. At this stage, it may often occur that when rising up from lying to sitting position, when laughing, coughing or leaning forward and in any other situation when the pressure in the rectum filled with gas exceeds the closing capacity of the sphincter muscle, intestinal gas escapes. It is also a sign of the weakness of the anal sphincter muscle when the underwear gets soiled during the day, in spite of proper daily cleansing. In the case of **rectocele**, defecation may often become difficult or painful. The emptying of the rectum may become imperfect; one may feel that his bowels have not been completely emptied after going to the toilet. It may also occur that one will succeed in completing defecation after several trials only, in smaller amounts. There is a higher chance of having constipation. In severe cases, there may be occasional **fecal incontinence** and sometimes the rectal prolapse protrudes through the anus.

! Those men who suffer regularly from constipation get much more frequently prostate inflammation, compared to the rest of the male population.

The rectal ampulla is a dilatable “sack” that can well adjust itself to the quantity of feces, capable of expansion within wide limits. Unfortunately, our everyday habits not only characteristic of our personal features, but also formed because of our life management regulated by artificial time limits, make us overexpand the tissues of this anal region. If we often hold back bowel movements (stool retention), delay going to the toilet in time, the waste material is kept in for a long time causing a stretching effect; therefore the bowel wall begins to adapt itself that is starts to stretch out. The lengthened section requiring more space may take the line of least resistance. If the anal sphincter muscle is weak, the dilated bowel section may protrude through the anus because of the slight resistance of the anal sphincter muscle. Internal hemorrhoids also may protrude (prolapse) outside the anus.

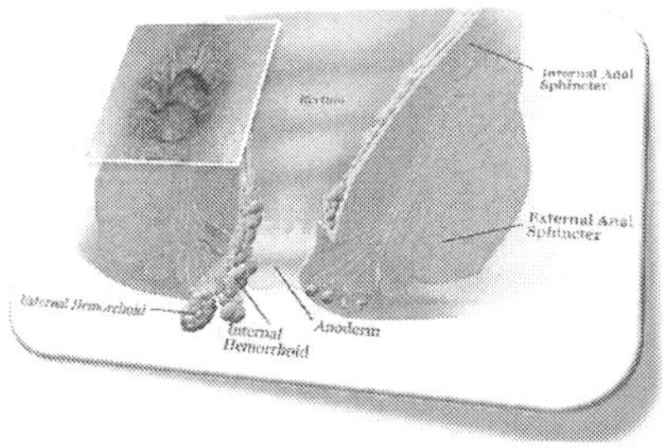

Hemorrhoidal plexuses are part of the normal human anatomy of the anal canal. They should not be considered pathological. These so-called arteriovenous pads are covered with mucous membrane and have the function to ensure a hermetic closure for the anus in all three dimensions. They become pathological when lengthened, swollen or inflamed and protruding outside through the anus. The person suffering from the symptoms of **hemorrhoids** will face sometimes stronger, other times milder troubles, discomfort. This means, the hemorrhoids are provoked by the subject himself some way. Hemorrhoids as disease, is a symptom of lifestyle adaptation. It has adjusted itself to those bad everyday habits by which we influence the perineal tissues. For example, we exert strength during sports; exert strong pressure in the case of constipation, do hard physical work... At a certain point, our body starts adapting itself.

Advices to preserve your intimate health

It is worth to follow these advices to preserve your intimate health:

We must take up with the idea that our body parts covered by underwear need care and bothering, too. Many ingrained habits, improper daily routines greatly contribute to the appearance and development of certain diseases, abnormalities. Such diseases include: stress incontinence, fecal incontinence, rectocele (rectal prolapse), predisposition to inflammatory disease in the pelvic region, hemorrhoids etc... The inappropriate habits regularly repeated for a longer time will bring along harmful effects. It is therefore expedient to change them for the sake of our health.

Defecation is also an everyday physical activity, therefore it is not indifferent when and how we do it. If we come to think it over how much time we spend in the toilet in a lifetime, it is easy to understand that if we burden or load ourselves in the wrong way in the meantime; it may surely become a serious risk factor for our pelvic floor muscles.

- It is important to wash hands before and after the use of the toilet. Prostatitis or cystitis among men is often caused by bacteria found on unwashed or dirty hands.
- Appropriate and regular defecation is very important. If you regularly suffer from constipation and the rectum is "filled up" too often and the rectal walls expand due to the fecal materials, filling it from within, the prostate may get under pressure and its blood circulation may be affected thereby. To avoid defecation to become a hard physical work, to produce normal-consistency feces, it is important to drink a suitable quantity of fluid. It can be understood that many people suffering from incontinence try to reduce the urine leakage by reducing the fluid intake. In fact, they are wrong in doing so. The human body needs water for the normal function, and its withdrawal may even worsen the state of incontinence. The urinary problems are not dependant on the volume of water intake. One of the most important roles played by water is to wash out the poisonous substances from the body – this is a process of essential importance from the aspect of fat metabolism, as waste materials get compiled in a very

short time. It is also a considerable fact that dehydration may be the cause of constipation, hard stool, chronic tiredness and headache. It is also important to consume an adequate volume of fluid to help the bladder get perfectly empty, which may prevent the multiplication of pathogenic bacteria in the urinary bladder.

- A peaceful, quiet breakfast setting the whole digestive system in motion and a cup of hot drink should never be missed, because a certain kind of tension present in the stomach in the morning, the digestive apparatus - in reply to the stimulus - will change to a quicker function and the intestinal system will strive for an early discharge following the meal. This is a natural reflex process not worth eliminating (gastrocolic reflex). It is a grave mistake to leave home in the morning without having breakfast or having just downed a small cup of coffee. Regular eating is indispensable to ensure a well-balanced intestinal activity and regular defecation as a result of that.
- During the day, we may be compelled by the circumstances to hold back bowel movements in spite of feeling a stimulus. When at home, this is less likely. The best solution would be, to get ourselves into the habit - even if afterwards, in adult age - of getting up 20 minutes earlier in the morning and going to the toilet and doing our job undisturbed, after having consumed some liquid. Holding back the urge to have a bowel movement may result in constipation. Those who have incontinence or recurrent prostatitis problem should pay even more attention to their digestion, since straining caused by constipation may do harm to the perineal musculature. If our body learns that we go to the toilet roughly at the same

time and under similar circumstances, defecation will be easy and almost automatic...

- Let's take care on consuming enough fiber, which will leave the body without absorption, and - constituting the decisive mass of feces – by exerting a significant pressure on the intestinal wall it will facilitate the cleaning of the intestinal system. Fibers are able to prevent constipation, but cannot do much good once the problem has already developed. Frequently occurs that one starts eating granola or oatmeal cookies, either at the doctor's advice, or just simply to increase fiber intake. This is very good for them in principle. However, one of the most frequent mistakes made in such cases is that people do not drink enough liquid simultaneously. Consequently, instead of improving digestion, constipation will rather develop. Oatmeal can absorb a quantity of liquid equals to 4 to 5 times their own weight; that is why it is important to increase the daily water intake in a similar rate. There is no benefit of eating fibers if you do not drink enough water at the same time to be absorbed by the fibers and help balancing defecation thereby. On certain occasions, when a bigger quantity of ballast materials is suddenly taken into an "untrained" intestinal system, intestinal gas formation may be provoked, resulting in unpleasant meteorism (trapped intestinal gas). Therefore, it is always suggested to adjust nutrition just step by step, and get the intestinal system used to the new nutrition habits slowly, gradually.
- The defecation stimulus signals the dilatedness of the rectum, the need that our body needs to get rid of the waste materials compiled. It is important that once we feel the stimulus, defecation should take place as soon as possible. In spite of this, many neglect and keep putting

off answering the stimulus for such a long time until it weakens and finally abates, and the waste matters remain in the body. Obviously, in many cases we are unable to go to the toilet in time, but it is no good regularly keeping the fecal materials, because the rectal ampulla can adapt itself to the storing need for a while - in a way that it gets dilated (rectocele may form).

- In order to keep the healthy state of the urinary bladder it is important not to keep storing urine for long periods. Having felt the impulse to urinate try to discharge urine as soon as possible. Observe the way you pee. It is important to pee with steady respiration, without exerting pressure. Pay attention and try to go to the toilet only when you have the express feeling that your bladder is filled up. It will have a worsening effect on bladder capacity if you keep on running to the toilet every now and then. Try to empty your bladder completely – this will be possible only if you wait with patience for the urine to exit. Even if you know the right way of urination, it will be expedient anyway to do a few urethral contractions after discharge, to help the urethra gets completely empty.
- It is important to ensure “free way” for stool. We should not sit in a stooped position even on the toilet, because the bowels get compressed that way and we should not force defecation with strong abdominal pressure, because that may contribute to the development of hemorrhoidal nodes. Discharge of stool should be carried out with an abdominal pressure as small as possible! Remember not to press or only to a very slight degree and for a short time. In the case of a normal stimulus and consistency of feces, normal and natural steady breathing - without any particular effort - is enough in itself. As mentioned before,

defecation by strain will make the supporting ligaments and pelvic floor muscles stretch out and lengthen accordingly. This is a similar physical work for the lower abdominal organs as if we regularly carried heavy weights. It is a generally known fact that frequent pressure is one of the eliciting factors of hemorrhoids. If you suffer from constipation, you may try to move the clod of feces out of its place. Try to move it out first, instead of pressure. So, you should make a movement as if trying to avoid passing gas or to hold back bowel movements, and after that press for a short while. If still, strain is unavoidable, the bodily position is very important. One of the best possibilities is to lean slightly forward, propping against our knees in order to avoid pressing the interior organs downwards. In this position, the weight of the interior organs will weigh on the abdominal wall instead of the perineum.

- After defecation, wash your genital area! It is worth always keeping a pack of wet wipes for intimate hygiene with you in case you are still unable to get washed. It does not occupy more place than a pack of tissue. Do not use rough of hard toilet paper to wipe your anal region, which may rub your skin around the anus sore and abraded, while not cleansing to the necessary extent. It is very important to use a separate towel to dry your genital region, not the same one as used for your hand. These towels should be changed much more frequently and hung out carefully after use - in order to get completely dry and avoid remaining wet or moist.
- It is important to protect the veins of the perineal region also after defecation. When defecation is finished, do a few medium-strength contractions with your anus to

restore normal blood circulation and muscular tone, then bend your trunk forward as if you wanted to touch your ankle, so that your bottom gets higher than your heart.

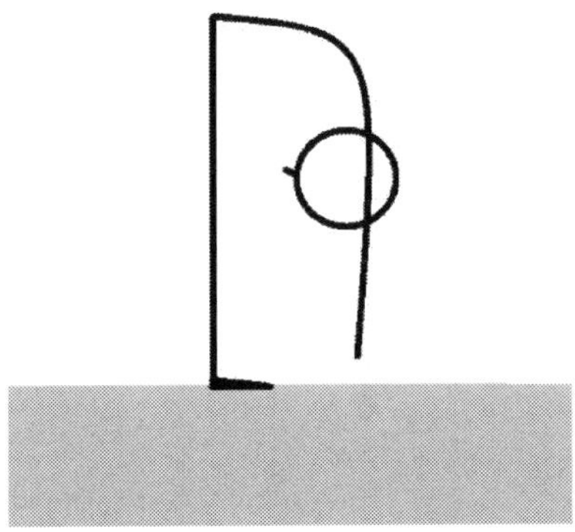

When – in a reverse bodily position – the pelvis is in a higher position than the heart, this helps the evacuation of deoxygenated blood from the perineal veins more quickly. This means that the blood filled with "waste" will be transported away from the pelvic region, and will be replaced by blood rich in oxygen and nutriments. The tension of the perineal muscles will cease as a result of the removal of the wastes. This is how you can assist venous circulation.

- The nutriment and oxygen supply of the tissues closing the pelvic floor can be improved by maintaining, keeping in good condition the blood vessels of the region. To reach that aim, it is advisable to rinse our genital region with cold water– after having the daily shower or bath- with a quick motion from the top of the pubic bone to the coccygeal vertebrae. The dilated blood vessels stretched out under the effect of warm water earlier will now strongly contract under the effect of the cold-water rinse. This is a kind of vascular fitness exercise, by which the nutriment supply of the tissues of the lower trunk may be improved.

- Physical work involving straining to lift heavy weights may also increase the intra-abdominal pressure. You should do physical work (lugging along, tiresome housework, sport etc.) only with an empty bladder. When the bladder is filled with urine, it exerts a heavy weight on the supporting ligaments, on the prostate and on the pelvic floor muscles, and if this is accompanied by strong abdominal pressure, too, it may result in the stretching of the supporting ligaments.
- You should avoid the consumption of any food or drink having an irritative effect on the bladder or prostate, or those causing worsening of the symptoms of prostatitis. These are for example the acidic food and drink, kinds of citrus fruits, spicy foods. The consumption of alcoholic drinks and those with a caffeine content should be reduced. Certain foods, fruit and vegetable juices – like tomato, melon, grape, pineapple or grapefruit – have an irritative effect on the urinary bladder, therefore it is worth reducing their consumption. The artificial sweeteners and hot spices should also be avoided.
- It is important to protect your bladder during a cough or sneeze when, if the bladder is filled, great load is exerted on the supporting ligaments. Simultaneously with coughing or sneezing, you can keep your bladder in a high position by contracting your pelvic floor muscles, avoiding thereby the injury of the supporting ligaments.

- The protection of the lumbar section of the spine is important to keep the ability of urinary continence and penile erection.

THE CONTROL TOTAL CONTRACTION - CT☑

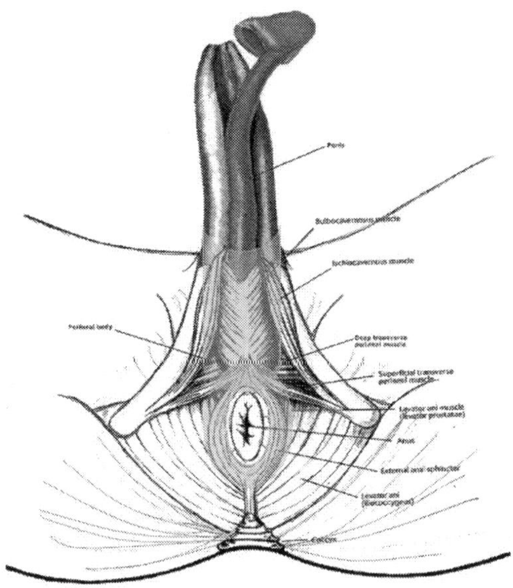

What is Control Total Contraction - CT☑ ?

You have already learned how to squeeze and relax the muscles around and in the penis, the anal sphincter and how to "lift up" the muscle region under the prostate. In the next exercise, you should tighten all the perineal muscle areas at once! You should feel that all the three muscle areas are moving according to your will. Even before all these three muscle areas were in operation; but now you should control the contraction of each section separately, to ensure that all the pelvic floor muscles should be adequately squeezed.

You have to check the contraction of all the three areas, because if you just squeeze and relax your pelvic muscles automatically, then the stronger sphincter muscle (usually the anal sphincter muscle) causes a stronger sensation, distracting your attention from your weaker sphincter muscle (or weaker part of the pelvic floor), consequently exactly the weaker sphincter muscle will not be squeezed properly and will not develop in the required way.

1. **In supine position with knees bent, feet flat on the floor. Relax your abdominal muscles. Perform an imitating movement of stool retention, as though you are trying to keep under control an urge of diarrhea or as if you are trying to stop passing gas. Right after perform an imitating movement of urine retention, as though you are trying to stop the flow of urine and parallel also try to "lift" the scrotum up. Through your mind, check the contraction of all the three muscle areas. If you are sure that you are actually squeezing all the three muscle areas, relax your pelvic floor muscles. Let your abdominal muscles become soft, make a slow elongated exhalation.**

2. **The next task is to perform a contraction of Control Total squeeze, just like before but with your maximum force, to provide enough stimuli to your pelvic floor muscles to induce muscle growth. To achieve this, you have to control consciously the**

closure of the two openings (anal and urethral) and the "lifting" of your scrotum. After the squeeze performed with maximum force, make sure that you relax all the three muscle areas properly. When you relax your pelvic floor muscles you should feel a sensation of "letting go". The pelvic muscles are imbued with a feeling of rest and relaxation.

3. **Now you should repeat the Control Total squeeze with all your force and holding the maximal squeeze for a count of 6, in the meantime observe yourself how you breathe!**

How did you breathe?

Most of the people, holding a strong muscle contraction, are not able to control their breathing. It happens often, that during the exhalation phase they cannot hold the muscle squeeze, their muscles relax completely or partially, although this is not their intention. To tell the truth, for the pelvic floor muscles is indifferent the way, how we take a breath during exercise, but if we would like to use our pelvic floor muscles in the everyday life, then it's very important to learn how to take our breath correctly, since coughing, sneezing, laughing and talking are all various forms of exhalation. Although a well-trained, strong sphincter muscle, due to the increased muscle mass, is closing well even without doing a squeeze with the pelvic floor muscles. However, there are some situations where it might be useful to increase the force of the closure of our sphincters, breathing normally. In case of “emergency” is an advantage, if you are able to hold the squeeze of your sphincters also during exhalation, in situations like having diarrhea or if you are forced to hold back urine, because you cannot find a toilet nearby. Thus, the purpose is not only to strengthen the pelvic floor muscles, but also to learn, how to control their function. You should also squeeze your sphincter muscles when you cough or sneeze, not only to prevent the unwanted urine leakage, but also to keep the pelvic organs in their proper place and to prevent the stretching of the supporting ligaments of the pelvic organs.

The importance of breathing correctly

Although you can squeeze your pelvic floor muscles voluntary, it is very important that your attention should remain on the functioning of the sphincter muscles till the end of the exercise / squeeze, because if something distracts your attention just for a moment, it may happen that the contraction of your sphincter muscle will be vanished suddenly. The squeeze of the sphincter muscle should not relax during exhalation. You are who squeeze and relax your pelvic muscles, whenever you want. Your pelvic floor muscles will be tightened only if you tighten them. It is very important to know that, when you want to hold the contraction of the pelvic floor muscles, you should breathe into your chest, because if you breathe into your belly, then together with the relaxation of the abdominal muscles, also your sphincter muscle will be relaxed. Do not worry, if you are still not able to divide your attention and make the pelvic floor squeeze independently from breathing. Exercising regularly at home you will learn the ability to keep contracted your muscles also during exhalation.

How to use the muscles of the pelvic floor automatically, in the daily life?

The following quite complex exercise will help you to learn how to use the muscles of the pelvic floor automatically, in all situations of your daily life.

! When you perform the Control Total squeeze, you should always follow closely with your attention the contraction of your weaker sphincter muscle, performed with maximum force. Then you can be sure, that both of your sphincter muscles will be tightened correctly.

In supine position with knees bent, feet flat on the floor. Start with a few abdominal breathing. During the inhalation phase, you should feel as your belly expand comfortably,

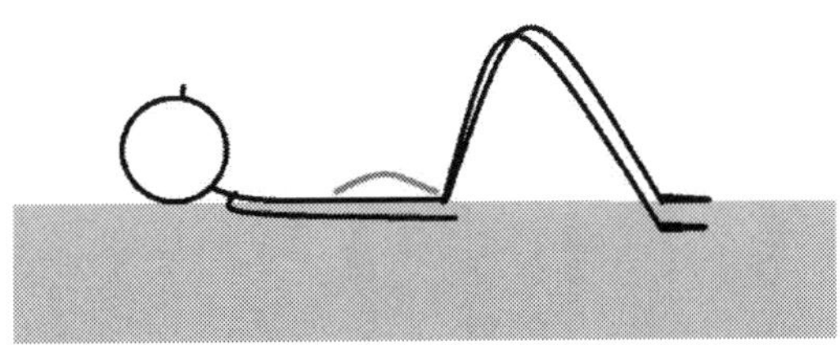

As you exhale press your knees against each other, perform a Control Total contraction with maximum force and as you exhale, holding the squeeze, lift your hips off the mat, still holding the squeeze, slowly lower your hips to the starting position,

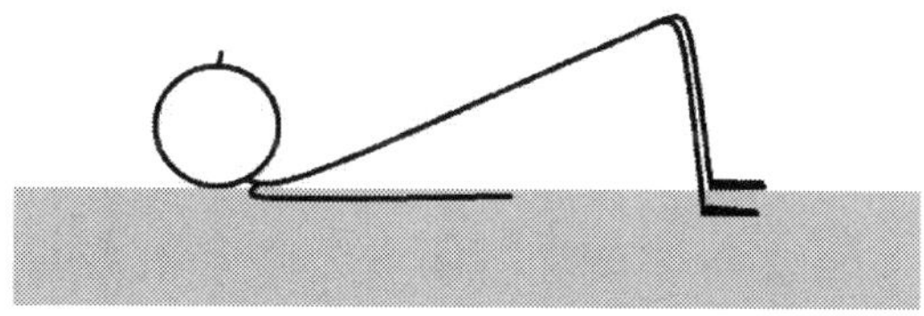

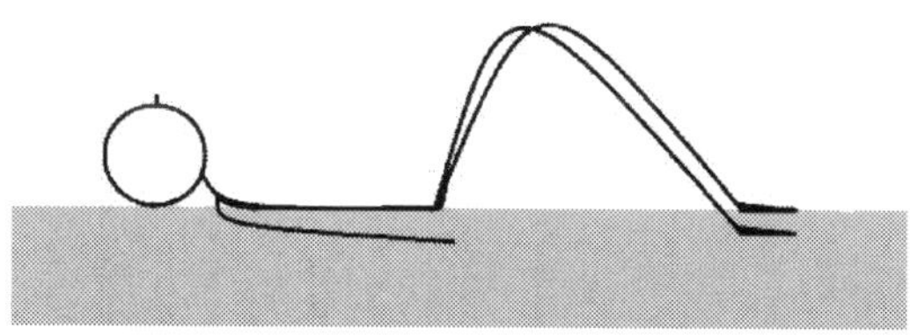

Still holding the Control Total contraction, raise your trunk up off the floor, roll back and relax. During the next inhalation phase, you should feel as your belly expand comfortably,

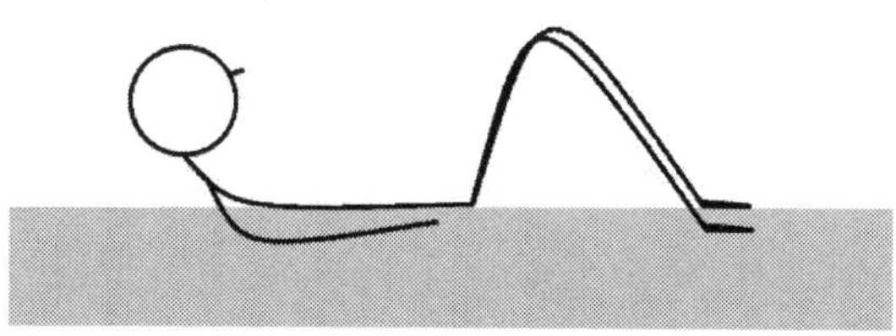

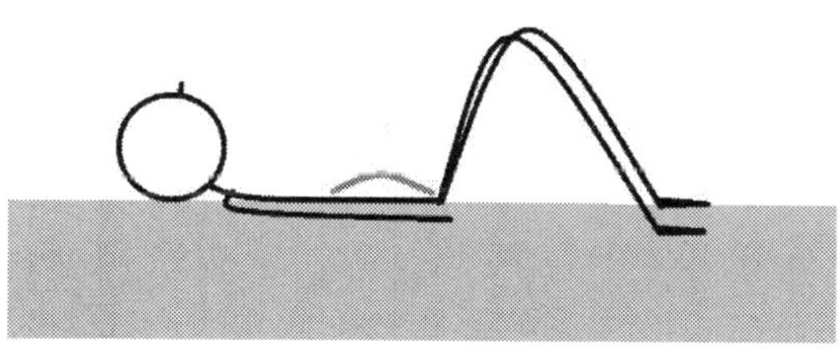

As you exhale perform a Control Total squeeze with maximum force, holding the contraction, begin to open up your knees apart, but only up to that point, where still you can hold the squeeze of the pelvic floor muscles, keep your legs in this position, begin to "waving" with your legs slightly apart 4 times (" little openings"),

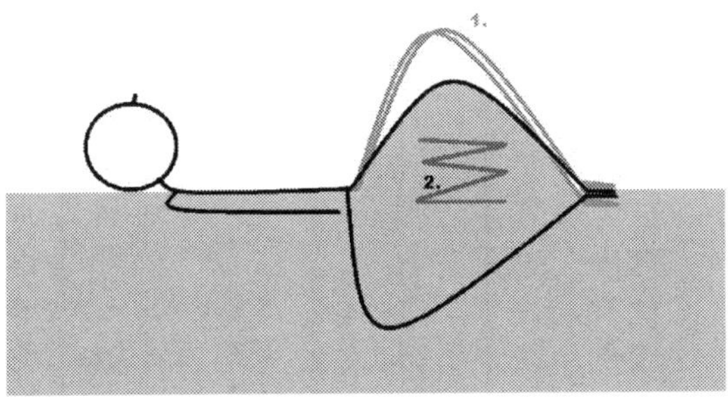

As you exhale, close your knees pressing against each other, during the next exhalation phase lift your hips off the mat,

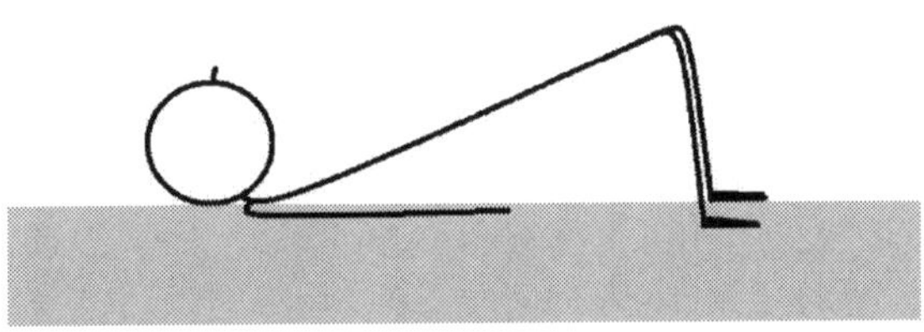

Still holding the Control Total squeeze, slowly lower your hips to the starting position, and relax your muscles, spread your knees as far apart as possible, let your abdominal muscles become soft, slow elongated exhalation. Perform 3-4 abdominal breathing.

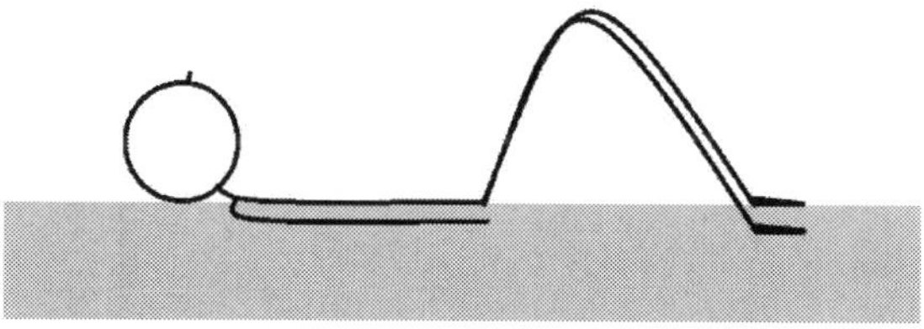

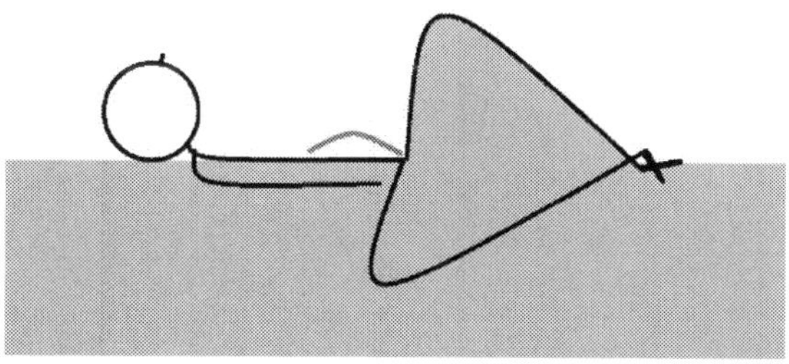

When you'll be able to keep your sphincter muscles squeezed in supine position, during exhalation, then you will be able to do it in any other posture and situation, for example, even when walking along the streets and you will need to sneeze or cough or meanwhile having sexual intercourse etc.

LIFESTYLE

How to practice sports in the right way?

Sport is a kind of physical exertion, therefore it is not indifferent, what kind of burdens or loads are affecting our body. Every kind of physical exercise has its internal effect as well. When one works for his health by doing sports (not in the proper way), it may have an effect just the opposite!

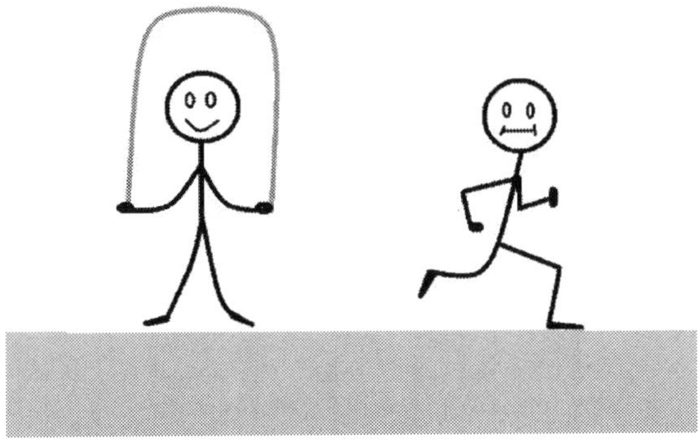

During skipping, hopping or jumping our internal body organs are similarly "skipping", exerting a heavy load on the supporting ligaments of the pelvic organs. For that reason, it is advisable to do this kind of exercise within reasonable bounds only. Running with incorrect technique is harmful to the lower abdominal organs as well as to the healthy state of the spinal column. If one insists on running, he must have the right running shoes and strong perineal muscles, right body posture and should try to run with the slightest possible bumps or shocks. Walking at fast speed will do no harm to anyone, while being similarly effective.

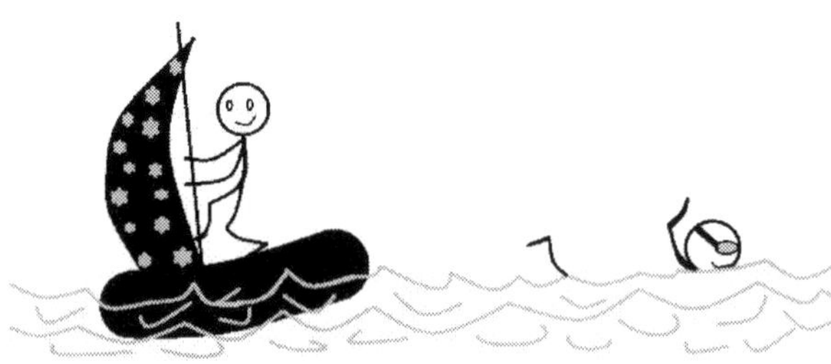

Always dry yourself properly after water sport activities and change into dry clothes, as wet clothes may cause cystitis, prostatitis, colds or fungal infections.

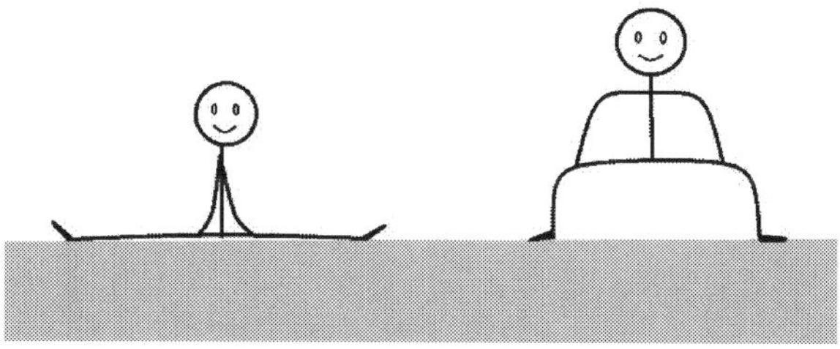

Exercises in a straddle – with legs wide apart – should only be carried out simultaneously contracting the perineal musculature!

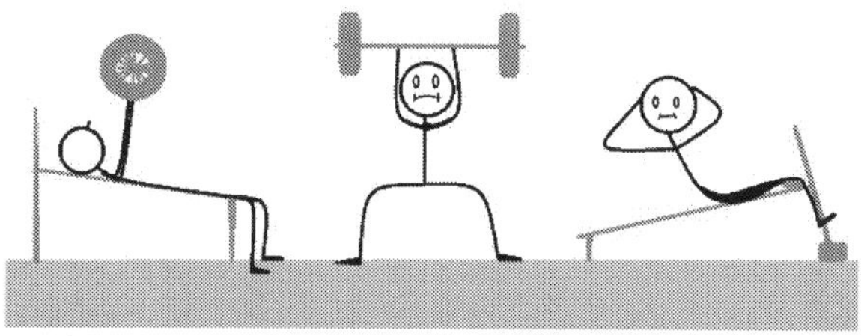

Gymnastic exercises carried out by pressure – whether in standing or sitting position – are similar in effect to the growing pressure occurring in the abdominal cavity during defecation by exertion. On such occasions the lower abdominal circulation slows down, the flow back in the veins takes place with difficulty. Hemorrhoids or testicular varicosity may develop as a consequence of strong pressures like that. These exercises should be carried out simultaneously squeezing the perineal muscles, lying on your back or side, or on all four position only, otherwise you may contribute to the descend of the urinary bladder or the rectum (especially after prostate surgery) – as a side effect of sport.

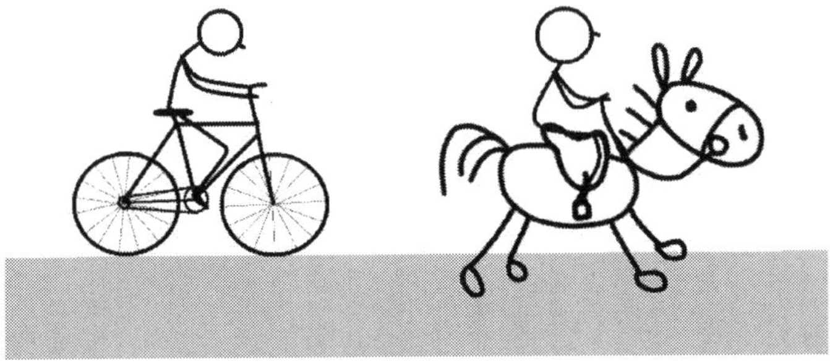

Riding a bicycle or a horse for longer period of time does not good for fertility or the health of the prostate. If you sit for more than half an hour continuously on the saddle (in a stooped position) and especially, if you wear tight bike pants, the temperature of the testicles may rise to an extent that will already affect negatively spermatogenesis. The numbness and insensibility of the pubic region, caused by the compression of the sensory nerves and arteries will be added to that. You should anyway choose a seat neither too hard nor too narrow and adjust it in a way so as to relieve the pressure exerted on the perineal region as much as possible. In addition to that, when riding a bicycle it is advisable to stop in every 30 minutes to have a break and do a few IWT® exercises (for example the Flipper exercise in standing position) and right after to position yourself in a reverse body position for a few seconds to increase muscular tone and restore the circulation of the perineal region.

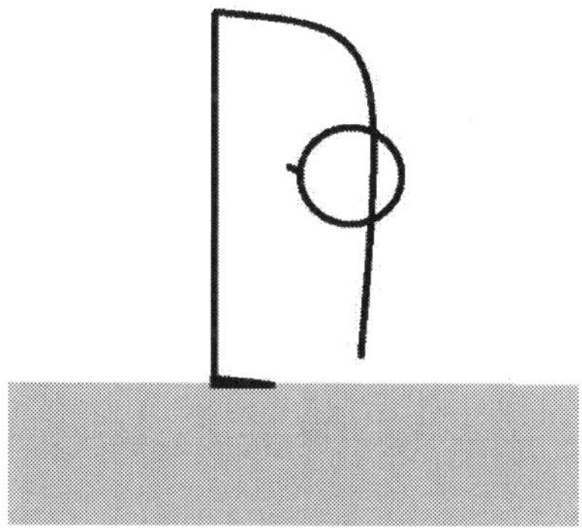

How to prevent the diseases of the prostate?

As long as the prostate works normally, causing no problem, no one would even think of it. However, sooner or later a significant part of men will have to become aware of its existence.

The prostate is a chestnut-shaped and -sized organ, located in front of the rectum, below the neck of the bladder and surrounds the urethra. The secretion of the prostate and the seminal vesicle fluid are equally needed for the movement and metabolism of spermatozoa. The prostate plays a very important role in fertilizing, as its secretion increases the semen volume and reduces its density. As a result of the contraction of the muscles of the prostate a certain fluid is squeezed during ejaculation, which is added to the semen. The size and function of the sex glands depend on the effects of sex hormones. Growing older, the quantity of male sex hormone (testosterone) diminishes in the male body, resulting in a relative predominance of the female sex hormone present in all men in a small quantity. This may induce the growing of the prostate, which phenomenon is called benign prostate enlargement, also called **benign prostatic hyperplasia** (BPH). It is the normal testosterone level that keeps the prostate within normal size limits.

Prostatitis, whether acute or chronic, may occur at any age. Its most frequent cause is a kind of bacterial infection coming from other regions of the body, such as first of all that of the teeth, the tonsils and the maxillary sinus, that may affect the prostate. It is therefore important to have the teeth and tonsils checked once inflammation has occurred. Recurrent prostate inflammation, if unattended or uncared-for for a longer time may even cause prostate cancer. However, a so-called nonbacterial prostatitis is often diagnosed too, in which no pathogenic agent is present. In this case, the prostate may simply have had an attack of cramp, but the cramp of the prostate does have its reason. There may be a blood supply deficiency, functional disorder of the smooth muscles or secretion problems in the background of the cramp etc... When, for example, the pelvic floor musculature is weak and the prostate is unable to "squeeze" its secretion, the stasis caused by that may result in inflammation. The cramps causing pain can be very well relieved with the help of IWT® exercises. It may also happen that pathogenic and "sterile" inflammations follow each other. Prostatitis may partially or even completely hinder urination i. e. the complete evacuation of the urinary bladder, which results in urinary retention. This will in turn, make the bladder more susceptible to infection, as the number of bacteria gradually increases in the retained urine; and then, the infection of the bladder may easily progress and extend to the urethra and the kidney. So, it can be clearly established that the prostate plays a decisive role in a great part of male urinary problems.

The following symptom complex is characteristic of prostatitis, benign prostate enlargement and prostate cancer as well: frequent urination (especially at night), difficulties in urination, weak flow of urine, emission of urine by drops, stinging, burning sensation during urination, shivering. Pain may be felt in the region behind the scrotum or painful ejaculation may also occur. If these symptoms present themselves, it is advisable to see a specialist.

The development of **prostate cancer** cannot be attributed to one single cause. The increasing risk of its occurrence is generally characterized by different risk factors, such as: elevated hormone levels, age, obesity, harmful workplace environment, diabetes and hereditary predisposition etc... Some of these factors can be influenced, some cannot. You cannot expect to be able to control all factors that have an improving influence on prostate cancer risk, but you can make certain steps for the good prostate health.

Many people think that there is nothing to do against hereditary predisposition: If – by expensive gene tests (DNA-based tests) – it is found that the healthy state of the prostate is endangered by a hereditary "gene defect", this finding should not be considered a death sentence. However, it is often not the deficient genes that are inherited, but rather the bad lifestyle habits, the unfavorable examples shown by the father. This is, for example, the case when the father who died in prostate cancer, used to show himself much stronger than he actually was. He tried to avoid emotional conflicts in his partnership this way. He may have possibly endured on a regular basis that his wife humbles him day after day. He may also have had a chronic constipation doing nothing against it or he had bad eating habits...

The sex organs are strongly affected by all psychological factors that have a negative influence on male self-respect. Prostate is the organ of male self-confidence. From the narration of many male patients, it can be established that in the background of their prostate problems there are: durable stress, strong force to achieve performance, injuries suffered in relation to their masculine self-respect or discontent with their own sexuality. So, it is important that men live their masculine role in an authentic way, without self-deception.

Age is another risk factor, against which men would not even think of doing anything! (Plastic surgery can help make improvements in your appearance but does not help in prostate cancer prevention!) If you come to think what does, an average man during the years to keep his prostate healthy, you will find nearly nothing! According to statistical data, the chance of the occurrence of prostate cancer is gradually increasing in line with ageing, but why? An average man never in his life would help his body get rid of the toxins piled up – by undergoing detoxification or purifying cures. He would not strengthen the muscles under the prostate by pelvic floor exercises, which would help evacuating the secretion of thc prostate gland and would improve its blood circulation. He stifles or holds back his real feelings, which causes emotional stress. Follows unhealthy nutrition habits, suffers from constipation, often sits or stands in a stooped position etc. Having reached a certain “stress level”, our body is unable to compensate any more the effects of the “sins” we commit against it. The environmental effects – everyday habits, traditions and wrong examples – have a greater influence on our life expectancy and prospects than inherited features. *But who is responsible for developing them?*

What can men do themselves for their own health?

Useful advices to prevent prostate problems and diseases

- If one has prostatitis, the fluid intake should be increased by drinking plenty of mineral water in order to urge urination, prevent urinary retention and renal infection.
- If you would like to keep or improve the health of your prostate, the birch leaves might be your best friend for the rest of your life. The infusion of birch is in fact one of the best herbal remedies for treating the urinary tract since it increases the production of urine 5-6 times more. The herbal tea with birch helps to dissolve kidney stones and sand, facilitating their expulsion from the body without pain.

  This is the way how you should prepare and drink the tea: Take 2 tablespoon of dried birch leaves and put them in half a liter of boiling water, wait a minute until it starts boiling again, stir and cover it. Let the tea stand for 20 minutes then strain it. You should drink all of the tea without any sweeteners, in less than 30 minutes, preferably in the morning hours. Do not forget to drink plenty of water throughout the day. You can do this cleaning cure once or twice a week.

  ! Birch leaves are high in salicylates, so if you have an aspirin allergy or sensitivity, the use of the infusion of birch is contraindicated because it can trigger an allergic reaction. If there is any doubt having an aspirin sensitivity, do not drink this herbal tea until you have spoken to an expert allergologist.
- In the case of prostatitis sexual activity may irritate the prostate and delay recovery, it is therefore suggested to moderate or avoid sex during that time.
- Magnesium has an influence on muscular tone, too, and helps in relieving the possible cramp of the prostate.

- I do not recommend rectal prostate massage ***for several reasons***, especially not with different manual devices. **1!** Prostatitis is often caused by inexpertly executed catheterization, cystoscopy or various unprofessional devices aimed at domestic use. It is easy to examine or massage the prostate through the rectum, because nothing but a thin wall separates it from the rectum. However, if the mucous membrane gets hurt there, the pathogenic agents of the rectum will get into the prostate through the lymph paths. **2!** There are two kinds of sphincters in the rectum. The inner one is continuously closed, whether during sleeping or working. This sphincter opens under the effect of the defecation reflex only, or in one other case: if, for example, it is forced to open or burst through by a great strength, e.g. an instrument or the doctor's finger on the occasion of prostate examination. If this sphincter is damaged or subject to regular widening or expansion, it will be able to stretch on a permanent basis, which may result in fecal incontinence. Unfortunately, it cannot be told in advance, how much load can one's sphincter muscle endure. We are able to exercise the external anal sphincter only, but the internal one cannot be voluntarily influenced. **3!** Prostate massage whether performed by a doctor or by various special aids can be exercised under given circumstances or in certain periods of time only. It depends on the doctor's timetable or your working hours, for example. No one will possibly walk around the office with massage devices inserted in his rectum.

Rectal Examination for Enlarged Prostate

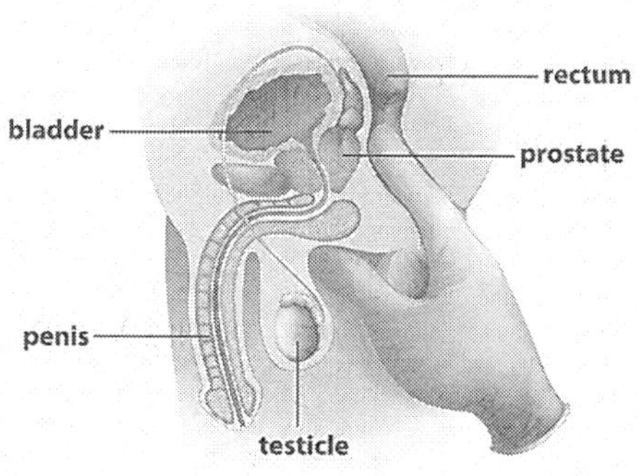

However, the correctly learned IWT® exercises can be performed even in office, even in every hour, without anyone noticing. Do not forget that the major goal in the case of prostatitis is to make the accumulating secretion leave the prostate as soon as possible. Another great advantage of the IWT® pelvic floor exercises is that men are able to adjust the intensity of the exercise as compared to the pain they feel, which is impossible during massage by the doctor.

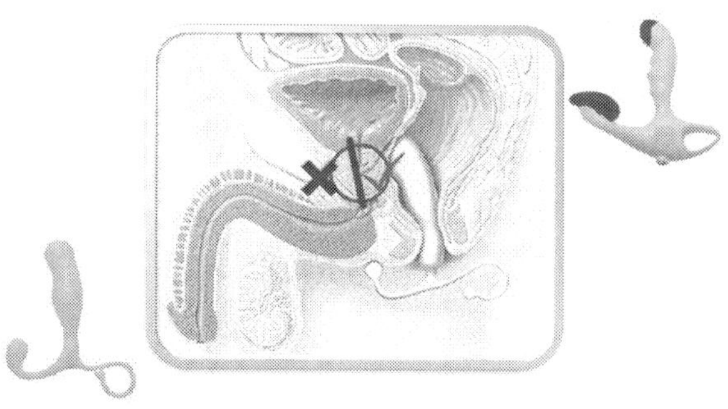

In addition to that, the doctor can only reach and massage the part of the prostate near the rectum, while with the IWT® pelvic floor exercises developed for this very purpose the prostate can be massaged all around, from all directions, resulting accordingly in a much rapid evacuation of the secretion and a quicker recovery, too.

S.O.S Exercise in case of prostatitis

When you have prostatitis, more times a day (even in every hour) when you have the possibility, do some steps in the upright position, then lift yourself on your tiptoes and lower yourself back down, do this rhythmically 15-20 times.

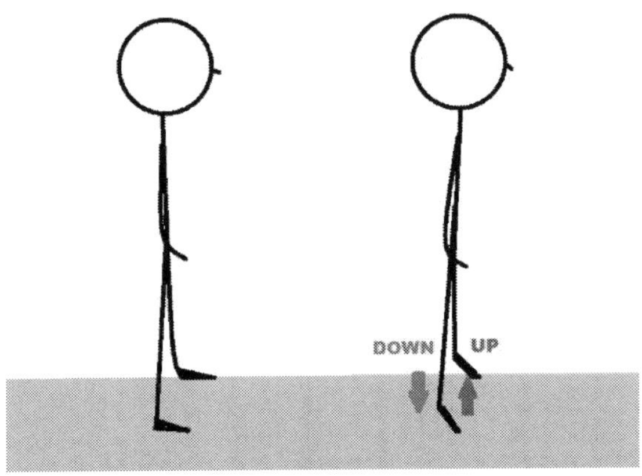

After this, 1-2 times perform the Flipper exercise, in any position, at any place (in the office, in the car, standing in front of a café automat etc.). Finally perform 8 short, fast, but strong Control Total squeeze, right after, position yourself in a reverse bodily position – when the pelvis is in a higher position than the heart, this helps the evacuation of deoxygenated blood from the perineal veins.

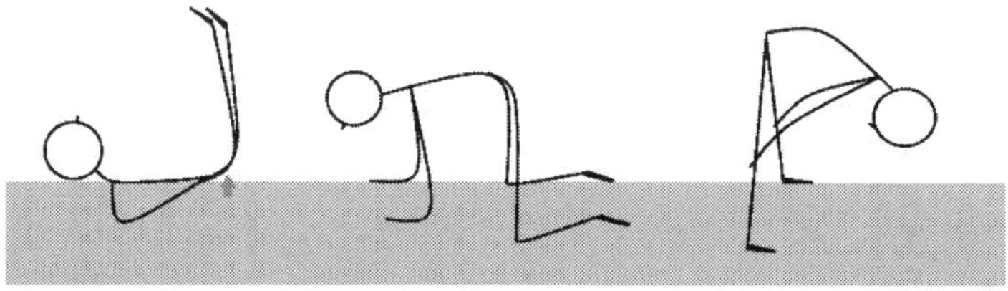

Obviously in your office not all of these the positions will be appreciated...

! Even if you do not have any problem with your prostate, it is suggested you to do this exercise every day to prevent prostate problems

- It is estimated that the major part of tumors start to develop slowly around the age of 20. However, the detection of cancer is generally happens around the age of 50 or later. Several studies show that turmeric can help in the prevention of prostate cancer and works also great as a complementary treatment. For example, in India, where an adult is consuming 3-5 grams of turmeric a day, all cancer rates are much lower than in western countries. Of course, in India besides the high consumption of turmeric, there are several dietary factors (such as vegetarianism) that may contribute to the lower cancer incidence rate. However, Turmeric has been tested in humans, in different clinical studies against various diseases with surprisingly good results. Turmeric, along with its uncountable positive effect, can help you fight bacteria and reduce risk of prostate infection. To prevent prostate problems I suggest you to take 1000 mg Turmeric supplement (only capsule form) daily. If you have prostate inflammation or cancer, you can increase the daily dose to 3000-4500 mg divided into three parts (breakfast-lunch-diner). (In clinical trials the daily consumption of turmeric was tested up to 8000 mg) However, you should be careful using turmeric if you have gallstones or bile duct dysfunction, if you are taking blood-thinning medications. In rare cases, extended use can cause stomach upset or heartburn, to prevent this you should take the capsules 30 minutes after eating. If you have questions about turmeric supplements, your pharmacist can answer many of them.

- Watch your weight! Both too much or too little fat stored may disturb the normal production of sex hormones and may also result in the reduction of sperm number and increase the rate of abnormal ones. Besides, if someone is obese, fat will be deposited not only externally, but also on the interior organs. The prostate is otherwise quite short of space, which will be even more cramped because of fatty layers, while deposits (plaques) formed by cholesterol will narrow the diameter of the blood vessels, resulting in a poorer blood supply of the prostate and the penis. Another important thing is that adipose tissue (fat cells) also produces hormones itself and may thereby disturb the quite sensible testosterone equilibrium, which may cause pathological enlargement or cancerous malformation of the prostate.
- Pay attention to your correct posture while sitting or standing! In the case of ideal posture the spinal column and the abdomen are preserved and kept by the muscles, accordingly the head is erect, looking straight forward, the back is upright – apart from its preserved natural double curve, the abdomen is flat, the pelvis leans forward with an angle of some 55-65 degrees.

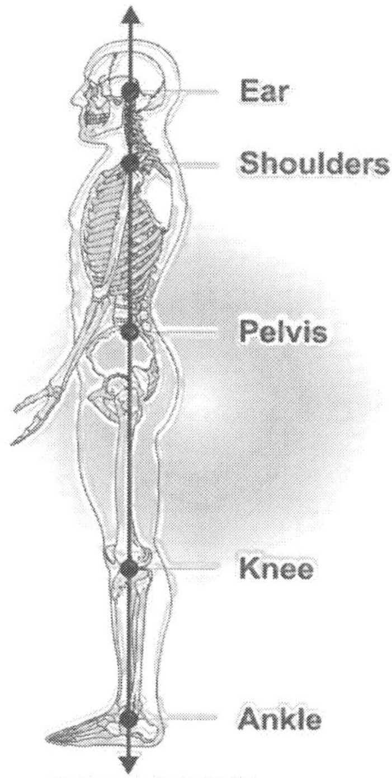

In the case of improper posture, the pelvis tilts forward at a greater degree, the abdomen bulges and the bottom shifts backwards. During sitting (especially in a stooped position, with possible constipation or with full bladder - to make it worse), the prostate is in a continuously compressed position, subject to a pressure both from underneath and from above. Its even so poor blood supply will further worsen, which may easily lead to inflammation. If – while doing durable sitting work – you do not forget to make your limbs stir and move for a while, the perineal musculature and the prostate will be relieved. Therefore, it is very important for a man to provide a more spacious place for his prostate. Stooped posture, dragging heavy weights with full urinary bladder, running, skipping, urination by strong abdominal pressure.

All these activities are increasing the intra-abdominal pressure or may weakening the supporting ligaments of the pelvic floor therefore may all have a harmful influence on the intact state of the bladder and prostate health.

- Mind your getting up in a way protecting the prostate, especially if the urinary bladder is full. On such occasions, the bladder presses against the prostate and weighs heavy on it. If you sit up from lying on your back, as if doing an abdominal muscle exercise, it will severely burden the supporting ligaments and pelvic muscles holding the bladder, since they will be loaded with the heavy weight of the urine. To perform a bladder-protecting uprising, roll onto your side and leaning on your arm, push your body to a sitting position.
- It is suggested - especially for those suffering from prostatitis - to reduce salt intake as well as the consumption of salty foods containing food preservatives. This can help avoiding water retention in the body. Try to rather use more herbs or aromatic medicinal plants in cooking or subsequent seasoning of food instead of salt. Raw food is a natural diuretic that, unsimilarly to drugs, fails to remove mineral substances from the body. The regular consumption of vegetables and fruits is very important to avoid constipation and painful defecation.
- Regular and too frequent consumption of meat may also have a negative effect on hormonal balance, since butcher's meat and meat products sold in the supermarkets contain plenty of estrogen and other hormones.
- A shower of the region of the perineum with cold and warm water by turns may have a very positive effect on prostate health (partial contrast bath therapy). Even if finding it unpleasant in the beginning though, you will feel

the favorable change later on. You should not "freeze" your penis, just have a short rinse of the perineal region with cold water.

- "Keep yourself cool...down!" If the temperature of the scrotum and the testicles rises, sperm production may be disturbed. Those who work in high-temperature places, wear tight-fit underwear, do a sitting work or just use their laptop keeping it on their groin, should count on the undesirable overheating of the testicles. It is highly recommended to avoid wearing tight underwear or trousers, to maintain good circulation in the pelvic area. Give up hot baths! Lengthy sitting in hot water may worsen sperm quality and quantity. More than half an hour spent in a water of 40 degrees Celsius (104 degrees Fahrenheit) will noticeably affect sperm numbers. The same can be said of sauna or steam bath, too.
- Zinc should be regularly topped up, since a great quantity is evacuated with sperm during ejaculation. Improve your diet with foods rich in zinc, that is eat more natural oily seeds, pumpkin seeds, brown rice, foods made of wholemeal cereals, but oatmeal, eggs and liver are also beneficial. You may ask why zinc is important? It plays a very important role in upkeeping the perfect function of the sex organs and the adequate level of sexual performance and vigour. It helps men to preserve the function of erection and contributes to the normal testosterone production and spermatogenesis. The decrease of zinc content has a negative effect on sperm motility first of all, while as a consequence of stress male gamete may lose its procreative ability. There is evidence that zinc may reduce the size of the enlarged prostate and the symptoms of prostatitis.

- Men have a soul, too, so their erectile dysfunction problem may also have mental causes. Emotional stress, repeatedly endured rejections, failures and criticism in office and at home will men devour and reduce their testosterone hormone levels. For that reason, it is inevitable to acquire the adequate stress management and relaxation techniques. Do physical exercise or sports regularly, as that can ease stress and help dissolve hormones inhibiting erection, but you should never go to the extreme, as that will do no good either! In men exercising themselves up to complete exhaustion, the normal hormone level will temporarily change, shifting blood pH to the acidic direction, which may worsen sperm quality, too.
- In line with ageing, exhaustion or fatigue, and regular sleep insufficiency may have an especially harmful effect on testosterone level diminishing anyway. Remember that if you generally miss the required average of 7-8 hours sleeping per day, the arrears cumulated during the whole week cannot be made up by sleeping until noon on Sunday, either from the aspect of testosterone or that of general health. A healthy prostate requires a normal testosterone level!
- Mind the toxins! As a result of environmental pollution, the increasing quantity of harmful substances in water, air and foodstuffs, the human body must perform a heavier work during detoxification. The various detoxification methods – fasting cures, purifying herb teas, infrasauna – can successfully stimulate the evacuation of "waste materials", residue and toxins piled up in the body, which not only improves the hormonal balance and strengthens the immune system, but also contributes to body weight

correction, too. A beginner in fasting should never start a cure longer than one day. Having faced and overcome the starting difficulties and having grown accustomed to the 24-hour cure, you may change over to the 36-hour one. It is most expedient to start on Friday evening, thus by Sunday noon you may have finished. (Severe headache can occur during fasting.) During that time, you must not consume anything but fluids: herbal tea, fresh fruit and vegetable juices, still mineral water. If you do not want to fast though, yet it is very useful to eat only fruits or vegetables once a week. This is the partial detoxification, which will greatly contribute to the normalization of defecation habits, too. It is forbidden to drink sweetened fluids (such as maple syrup) during fasting! Candida albicans (yeast – fungal organism) is present in the body of all human beings, without causing any problem, normally live on the skin and in the mucous membranes of the human body. We live in symbiosis with this organism from birth; its presence is absolutely part of the upkeep of normal intestinal flora. Its quantity is regulated by the benign bacteria promoting digestion, present in the intestinal tract, but if our immune system weakens for some reason, the fungus Candida Albicans may – though not in all cases - launch an attack. How can it become harmful? Improper nutrition, overblown intake of antibiotics, taking of contraceptives (as referring women), stress, mental and psychic problems may result in the reduction of the number of bacteria responsible for balance, providing very favorable conditions for the proliferation of the fungus. Sugared food, soft drinks or yeast-containing foods – all serve as hotbed for Candida infection. Fungal infections – contrary to public belief –

may occur not only among women, but among men and children, too. It is a hard job to confirm the presence of Candidiasis (yeast infection caused by the abnormal proliferation of yeast/Candida albicans). The generally applied method is to isolate (by cultivation) the pathogenic agent from the smear, discharge or feces. However, Candida is present in healthy organisms, too, it is therefore difficult to find if it has proliferated in the body to a pathological extent or only the fungi normally present have multiplied on the culture medium. The natural acid-base equilibrium is of decisive importance in the human body. In most cases, we do not even think that the disturbed acid-base equilibrium may be hidden in the background of various diseases. Overacidity is characteristic of the people of our age, mostly caused by improper nutrition (preserved foods, extreme consumption of meat and meat produce, black coffee, alcohol, protein, insufficient consumption of fruits and vegetables, inadequate chewing, inadequate consumption of liquid, exaggerated consumption of sugar and carbohydrates...), but other lifestyle and environmental effects may also have an influence on this indicator. The most common ones of them are smoking, the unreasonable and exaggerated slimming cure, lack of exercise, stress and excessive alcohol consumption. Extreme physical loading or overblown sport activities may also result in a shift towards acidity. The acid environment provides a favorable seedbed for diseases. In line with growing acidity, inflammatory processes are strengthened, while long-term performing capacity is reduced. The person soon gets exhausted and has a worsening disposition. As a general rule, to reach an optimal acid-base equilibrium in the human body, alkaline foods should be in about 80% predominance. If one consumes food of vegetable origin only, it is a great step towards alkalizing, but still cannot guarantee an adequately alkaline organism, because he/she may eat more than necessary, may eat more often than necessary, or may eat wrongly matched types of food. The most important thing is proper nutrition!

- Antibiotics (for example to treat prostatitis) and steroids destroy the essential intestinal flora and allow an overgrowth of the fungal yeast. Today it is generally known that the colon is responsible in some 70 - 80 % for the condition of the immune system. Therefore, the effective functioning of our immune system is subject to the condition of our intestinal tract - in 2/3rd part. Over acidity and overgrowth of fecal residue and plaque in the bowels may paralyze the immune system, which makes it more susceptible to certain infections that could be otherwise easily overcome by an intact immune system. This means: it is not the viruses and harmful bacteria that make us ill, but our overburdened immune system unable to cope with them. To restore the normal balance of intestinal flora and to help its proper function, you should take - 2 times a year for 2-3 weeks probiotic supplements (Lactobacillus acidophilus). Ask your pharmacist, for advice. (To eat yogurt is not enough for restoring normal bacteria in the intestine).
- To take Vitamin - C is always a good idea since it is a well-known antioxidant, expert in strengthening the immune system and helps to overcome stress and diseases. Vitamin - C also stops the growth of E.- coli, the most common bacteria involved in bacterial prostatitis. In case

of prostatitis, take 1000 mg Vitamin - C daily for 4 - 5 days.

- Smoking has a negative influence on the number and motility of sperm. Since nicotine has a vasoconstrictive effect, too, it will significantly reduce the capacity/intensity of penile erection.
- Excessive alcohol consumption greatly increases the chance of developing erectile dysfunction (ED). It is widely known that the desire of drunk or even just tipsy men is much bigger than their actual performing capacity. Drinking too much alcohol can lower testosterone levels and cause decreased sperm production, too.
- Keep off all kinds of drugs! Marijuana may reduce the number and motility of sperm, simultaneously increasing the rate of abnormal ones. The use of Cocaine and opiates is often accompanied by erection problems, while amphetamines may cause loss of libido.

The rules of male intimate hygiene

One side of the coin: the calvary of recurrent gynecological infections and their related treatments. No matter how prudent is a woman to her personal hygiene, she is forced to return to the gynecologist again and again because of the "ping-pong" infections. The vagina is located within the body, isolated from the outside world, its anatomical position may explain the late detection of any infection and at the same time, can provide favorable conditions for the proliferation of pathogenic bacteria. The other side of the coin: men's intimate hygiene, yet there can be serious deficiencies in its field today. The harmony of sexual life can be repeatedly ruined if during the intimate relationship the female partner is a victim of recurrent vaginal infections.

The opening of the male urethra is relatively distant from the anus, so the infections of the male urethra and genital area are not related to diseases in the same way as in case of women, since vaginal infections mainly are coming from the direction of the anus. Nevertheless, it is very important to respect the standards of male intimate hygiene.

How to keep your penis clean? - The prevention of unpleasant genital odors…

Many men neglect to clean thoroughly their penis despite that, the intimate hygiene is important to prevent diseases of the genital area. The hygiene of the penis becomes especially important before and after sexual intercourse or after masturbation.

If you are circumcised, all you need to do is gently wash the penis with warm water each time when you are having a shower or bath and rinse then dry it afterwards. Make sure you are using clean, dry towels every time you step out of the shower.

If you are uncircumcised, you will need to pull the foreskin back from the head of the penis to wash underneath. You should only pull your foreskin back as much as is comfortable, do not force it.

Rinse well the head of the penis and underneath the foreskin and then pull the foreskin back in place over the gland.

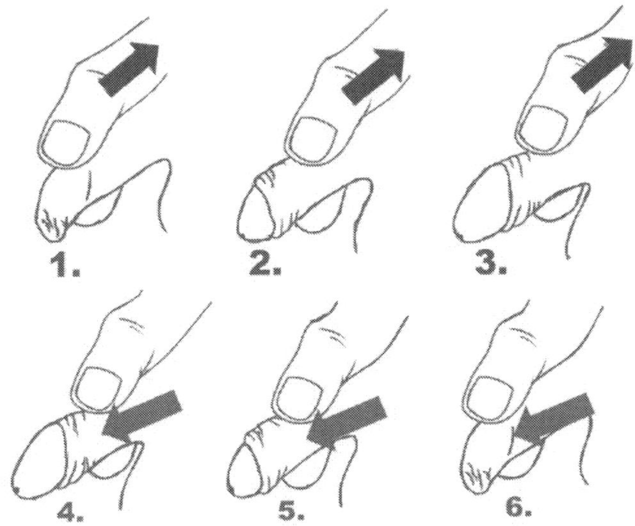

The secretion produced by the glands called smegma, placed in the glans under the foreskin; it helps the penis to penetrate the vagina and to ensure that the foreskin can easily slide on and off the head of the penis without irritation. Since the cheesy secretion of glands is rich in fatty acids, they are very good breeding ground for the bad bacteria. Both circumcised and uncircumcised men can develop smegma, however it will accumulate faster in uncircumcised men due to the foreskin. If the area under the foreskin is not kept regularly clean, may become the starting point of a very painful infection.

Prolonged bacterial infections may lead to severe chronic inflammation - even with no symptoms- of a part of the interior genital organs (prostate, Cowper's glands) – reaching these organs through the urethra. To prevent male urethral inflammation, it is very important to pull back the foreskin and clean the glans properly every time when you take a bath.

☝ Studies show that women value a man's personal hygiene much more than his penis size…

While regular personal hygiene is important, too much washing with detergents can cause irritation. It cannot be emphasized enough the importance of using a pH-neutral shower gel for intimate care. To clean the penis is not recommended to use aggressive soaps which may dissolve the protective layer on the thin surface of the glans, decreasing its resistance to infections.

Do not forget to clean also the base of the penis by the testicles and the area between the base of the testicles and the anus where sweat and hair can combine to produce an unpleasant strong smell. It is also a good idea to check your testicles once a month after a warm bath or shower. Furthermore, even tight pants and underwear made of synthetic fibers can create the "friendly environment" for various pathogens, therefore, it is recommended to use loose cotton underwear. Appropriate and regular disinfection of the toilet is essential.

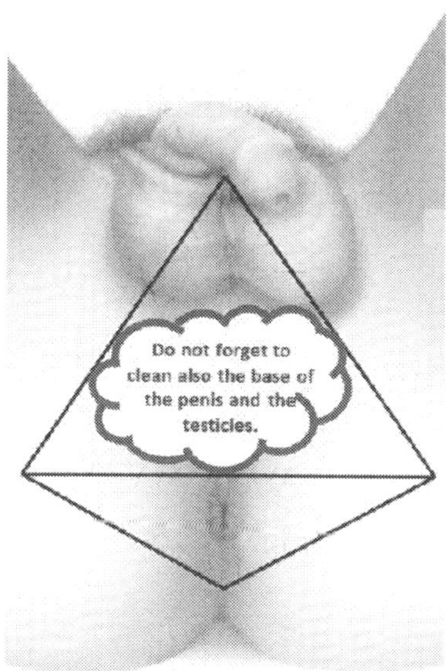

The genital organs of a part of men are infected with the HPV virus (Human Papilloma Virus) but in their case, usually it does not causing visible symptoms and the disease does not manifest itself. In women, the HPV virus - because of histological reasons - penetrates more easily into the deeper layer of epithelial tissue cells that covers the surface of the uterine cervix, which allows the virus to survive and proliferate. It is important to know that men are "carriers" of the risk of reinfection it means if a man infected from the HPV virus, may re-infect his partner who has recovered from her illness, whether vaginal or oral sex is involved. It is therefore suggested that a man whose partner is subjected to therapy with cervical cancer or in precancerous condition, to make a test to determine if he is infected or not by the HPV virus.

One more very important thing - Urine leakage after urination...

Losing a few drops of urine after you have finished passing urine is common in men of all ages. Many men find that even after waiting and shaking the penis, a bit of urine will leak out afterwards. This may happen if the urethra has not emptied completely and a small amount of urine gets left behind.

The male urethra is about a 15-20 cm long tube, which you pass urine through.

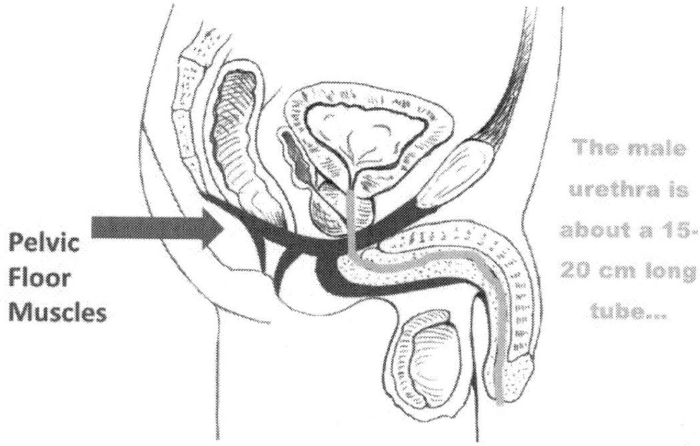

It is not enough to just shake the penis a little bit. Try to empty your bladder completely – this will be possible only if you wait with patience for the urine to exit. After you have finished passing urine, try to do a few light and fast urethral contraction by tightening your pelvic floor muscles. This movement will push the urine out of the urethra and help to stop the urine leakage.

Alternatively, after you have finished passing urine, wait a few seconds and then pull the foreskin back from the head of the penis after that, with a piece of folded toilet paper dry the penis gland, than from the base of the penis, gently move your fingers forward toward the head of the penis and keep pressing gently. This should push the urine further along the urethra.

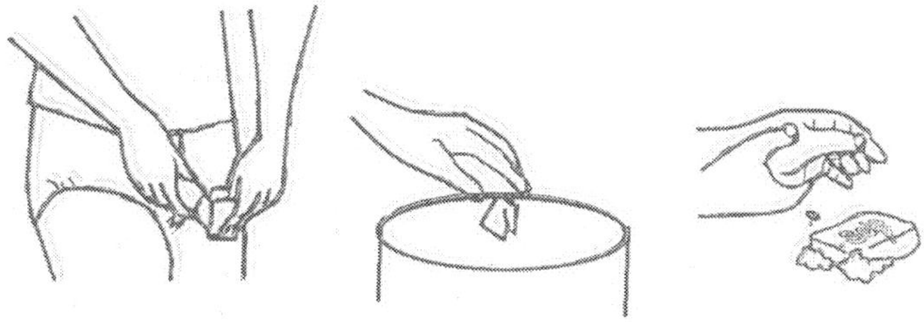

Also in this case you can do a few light and fast urethral contraction by tightening your pelvic floor muscles, after that shake the last few drops of urine out and let it to absorb with the toilet paper.

Do not forget to wash your hands after using the toilet!

Erectile Dysfunction (ED)

In spite of sexuality being discussed more and more open and straightforward nowadays, the majority of men feel ashamed having problems in bed, therefore they are rather silent about it. This reaction is related – among others – to the general delusion still alive in public that erectile dysfunction is equal to impotence. However, this latter refers to complete inability to erection, while erectile dysfunction means that a man is unable to reach or maintain an erection sufficient for satisfactory sexual performance. The development of erection requires a sexual stimulus on the one hand and a well operating vascular system on the other. Sexual arousal in itself is in vain if the system fails to work properly. Many people do not bother about having a higher blood pressure or having put on some weight, but failure in bed will definitely urge them to consult a specialist for help.

Potency disturbances may be generally classified in the following main groups:

- ***Organic*** – these are concomitant symptoms of organic changes and, by curing the basic disease they generally improve (if they are not too severe or not existing for a very long time) or may completely recover;
- ***Psychic*** – caused by a certain psychological block; (for example: unconscious fear of having a baby; sexual remorse rooted in childhood or education; fear of private situations, intimacy; if a man lacks success in his job or

profession or should face a challenge bigger than he is able to cope with, his sexual performance may decline as a result of stress...)

- ***A blurred mixture of the first two ones***, or a temporal transition between them, with one or the other coming to the front from time to time.

The leading cause of temporary potency disturbances has been stress and anxiety even today. In the animal world, stress is generally lifesaving. However, in human physiology it may be the cause of several diseases, and may even develop without an external harm. It always depends on individual features, what will generate stress in a given case, under the given circumstances. Today, when the weekdays of people are determined by the struggle for life (meaning: job, position, salary, promotion, mother-in-law, children etc.), women get frigid and sterile, while men suffer from premature ejaculation or erectile dysfunction.

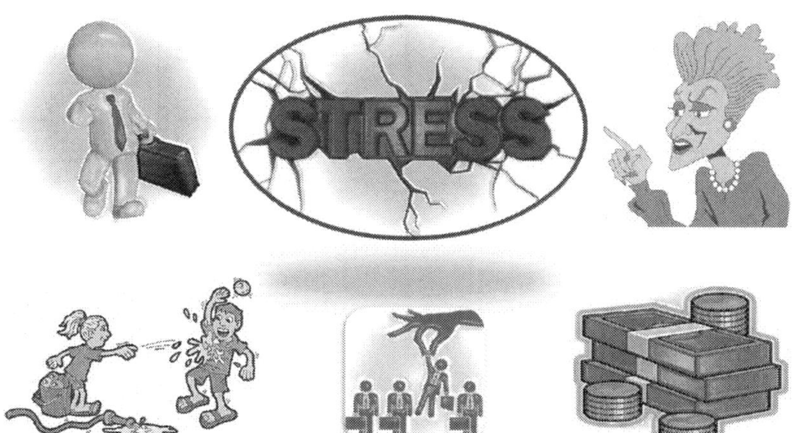

Premature ejaculation is general among anguished men. Potency is subject to relaxedness. If you are overburdened in both physical and mental sense, your body will start striving for relief. If, for instance, a man is tired, it is impossible that his penis alone can be fit and vigorous.

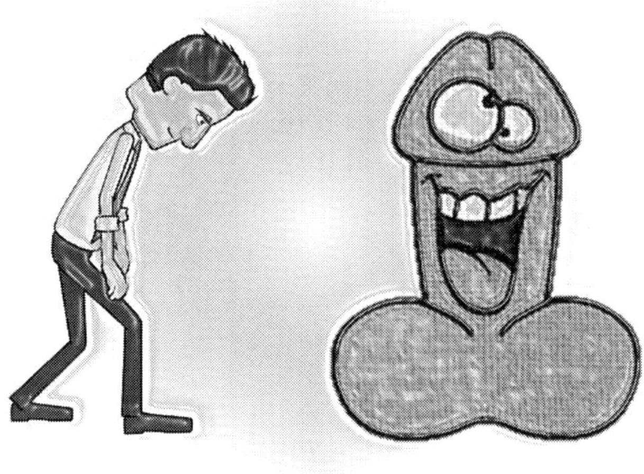

The condition of the body and musculature is always similar to that of the whole person. As internal state of mind changes, it will determine thc function of the sex organs, too. A sexologist once said it: I have never seen an escaping antelope with an erected penis.

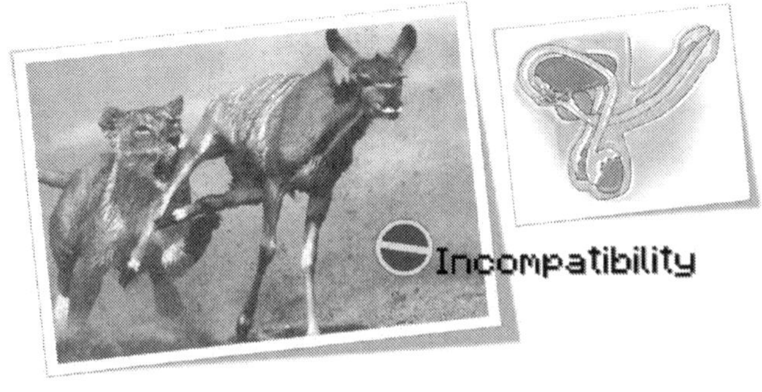

It is indifferent, what causes the man's escaping state: exhaustedness, stress, job problems. Your interior / mental health condition will always have a physical consequence. If a well-balanced interior mental state is not reached, no one pelvic floor exercise or gymnastics will make your sex organ work properly. The penis is very sincere and "tells you the truth". It cannot be erected voluntarily "against his will". It always reflects your actual state of mind. Your penis will not behave as a "good guy" down there, even if you try to pretend that everything is all right. The point is that human body is very clever: sometimes it shows the things disliked by the human psyche or body, the person himself being unaware of it. It is very important to accept that men are not push-button structures as a coffee-automat. You just press the button and you get the coffee (erection). There are certain conditions in which the body protects you with the **erectile dysfunction (ED)**. There are certain states of mind that are incompatible with male potency. Nature rejects supporting erection, as that would kill the person, in the case of certain diseases, taking medicine or overstressed physical or mental state for example. In spite of that, many men force their penis "to work" by taking Viagra. Well, body may perhaps adjust itself to that for a while, but then comes a heart attack. A little rest and stress management would do much more good to men.

Things worth knowing about premature ejaculation....

What does premature ejaculation mean? Early ejaculation – compared to what? – you would rightly ask. There may be certain differences of opinion even among andrologists and sexologists in defining the time considered premature ejaculation.

When a man complained of premature ejaculation to a well-known sexologist, she asked back: Tell me, sir, do you wet your pants, too? No, he answered shocked by amazement. Then the sexologist asked: And what do you do to avoid wetting yourself? Now, think it over, what is the way you do it! Men generally say on this occasion that when they feel the impulse to urinate, they hold it back. Sexologist: And why do you not do the same before ejaculation? The answer to this question is generally the same: Well, but how?

To control ejaculation is a similar function as that of urination. However we do feel the impulse to urinate, we relieve ourselves only when the circumstances so permit, or when we choose to “let it flow”. The control of ejaculation needs a learning process, but some get stuck at a point when they can only realize: gee, sperm has come off again. Adult men should be able to reach the stage in this learning process when they know what to do to avoid premature ejaculation.

Be present during sexual activity!

A man can be considered “professional” in controlling his ejaculation if he can stop at the point when he is on the edge of reaching that certain “nearly good” feeling. At this point, he can control ejaculation as much as he wants. However, if he is not completely concentrating on the act, but wonders if the children are listening, or thinks that the other woman was much better in bed than this one, or that had bigger breasts and this has small ones, in short: if he does not concentrate his attention to the current action, he may fail to notice in time that he approaches the “nearly good” point. Ejaculation and orgasm do not happen at the very same time, only if the man is in a big hurry. If he is not rushing, he may notice that these are to separate points. He should practice in the technique to identify that certain “nearly good” feeling (by masturbation). This is the clue of being able to prolong an act as long as he wants.

In learning the practice of IWT® exercises, you have to pay attention to slight internal sensations (when the sphincter muscle moves just slightly...). During sexual intercourse, the task is the same: pay attention to slight internal quivers and sensations. You should be aware you have reached the point in order to decide if you would like a long sexual intercourse, or wish to finish soon. Of course, it may also happen that the man wishing to prolong the act, he stops his rhythmic movements to delay ejaculation or pulls out his penis but his partner continue to move (that is a kind of stimulation, too!) and in the same moment semen spurts out of his penis. It was a good decision to stop the movements, but was a wrong action. Men should also learn to do the right action following a right decision. This is very important, because sexual self-evaluation determines the way a man feels himself in his own skin. A man can learn how to control ejaculation very soon, if his attitude is positive enough. All right, I did not succeed this time, next time I will take more care. If you are full of anxiety, you will not be able to learn it.

A few techniques for controlling premature ejaculation

- When the man feels ejaculation approaching, he should press on the penis right under the glans (head) with three fingers, until the sensation "ejaculating immediately" stops. He should maintain the pressure to last until the immediate urge for ejaculation ceases to exist. The clue of this stopping method is that the male should recognize the very moment after which he will not be able to control ejaculation any more.
- Another method of the stopping method is when feeling the approach of "the point from where there is no withdrawal" the male presses on a point with his left thumb and forefinger between his anus and scrotum (prostate point) for 3-4 seconds.

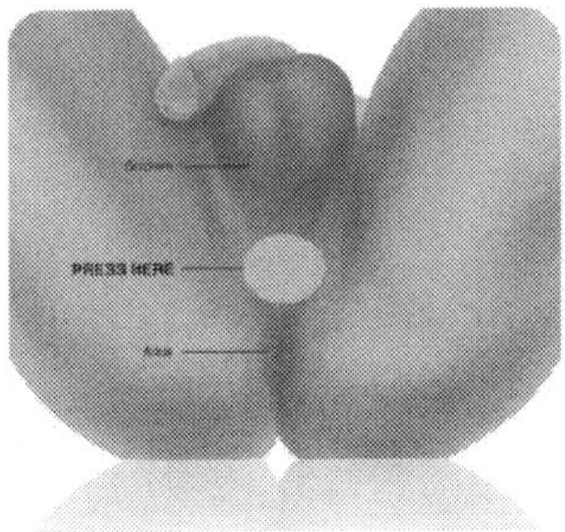

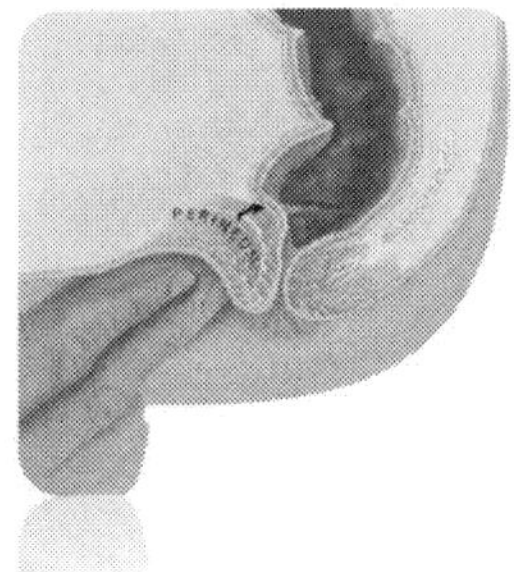

At the same time, he should take a deep breath. In this case, the penis should not be withdrawn from the vagina, but both partners should stop for a while! You may gently make your partner stop without telling her verbally. One, who has learned the correct technique of IWT® exercises and strengthened his pelvic floor muscles, will be able to control his ejaculation even without manual pressure, only by squeezing strongly his pelvic floor muscles ("lifting up" the prostate point).

- Finally, when a male feels ejaculation approaching, he should simply pull back his penis for 10 – 30 seconds. This way he can avoid the spurt out of semen. After that, he may penetrate again and go on with the sexual intercourse. The ability to keep and prolong erection also depends on the strength of the pelvic floor muscles: the stronger the pelvic floor muscles, the more vigorous and powerful the erection will be.

ADVANCED WORKOUT PLAN TO THE EVERYDAY PRACTICE

Balance scale exercise:

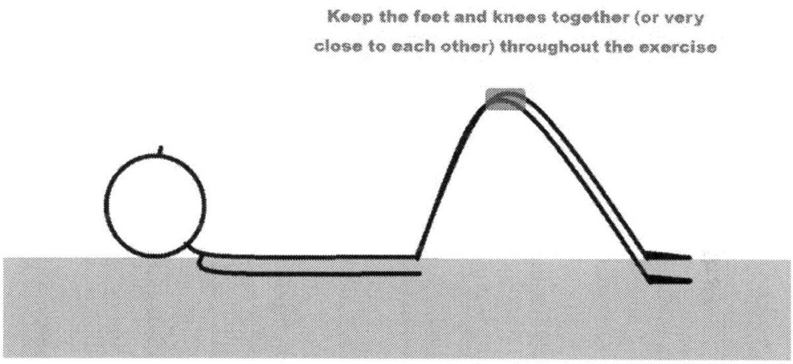

Part A: In supine position with knees bent, feet flat the floor (close to each other). Relax your abdominal muscles. Pay attention only to the muscles around and in your penis. Squeeze the muscles around your penis just a little bit, hold this slight tension. Move your pelvis forward, in this position there is a small "bridge" under the lower back. Increase the force of the contraction of the muscles around and in your penis till your maximum force; squeeze your penis tightly, try to "lift" the scrotum up as high as you can, "pull back" the base of your penis toward the rectum. Hold the squeeze counting to 6; squeeze the penis in its full-length. As you exhale, slowly, counting to 4, relax your penis muscles. Let your abdominal muscles become soft, perform a slow elongated exhalation. Allow the spine and pelvis to return to their original – neutral position.

Before continuing the exercise take a break counting to 5.

Part B: Relax your abdominal muscles. Pay attention only to the sphincter muscle ring around your anus. Squeeze slightly the muscles around your anus, hold this slight tension, move your pelvis backward – simultaneously tighten your buttock muscles and press your lower back down into the mat, increase the force of contraction of your buttock till the maximum force, squeeze the muscles around the anus as strongly as you can. Hold the squeeze counting to 6. As you exhale, slowly relax your muscles. Let your abdominal muscles become soft, make a slow elongated exhalation, almost like a sigh of relief. Allow the spine and pelvis to return to their original – neutral position. Before repeating the exercise, take a break counting to 30.

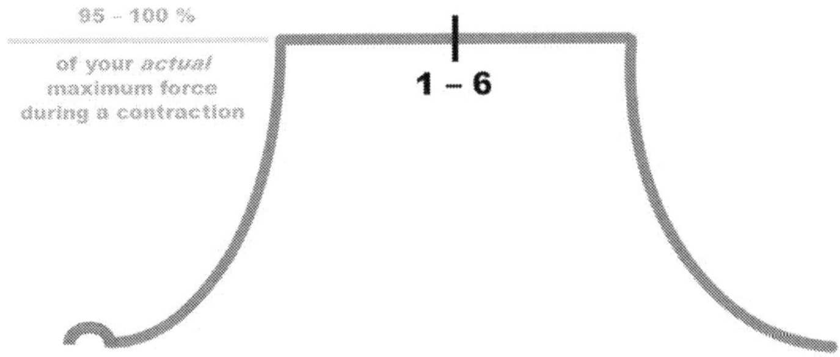

At the end of the repetitions of the exercise **(Part A-B)**, one time, perform 8 definite, short, fast and strong contraction alternately with your muscles around and in the penis and anal sphincter muscle, as quickly as you can. Do not try to hold on to the contractions, just squeeze and relax. Remain in supine position, with knees bent. In order to maintain a balance, place your arms on the floor alongside your body, palms facing down. As you exhale press your feet into the floor, slowly lift your pelvis up off the mat into a bridge, your pelvis is in line with your shoulders and knees; hold this position for 10 seconds. Remember to breathe! Release and roll slowly back down to the floor. Inhale deeply through your nose into your abdomen and slowly blow out the air while you relax your pelvis completely.

Perform 8 definite, short, fast and strong contractions with your actual pelvic floor area, as quickly as you can. Do not try to hold on to the contractions; just squeeze and relax.

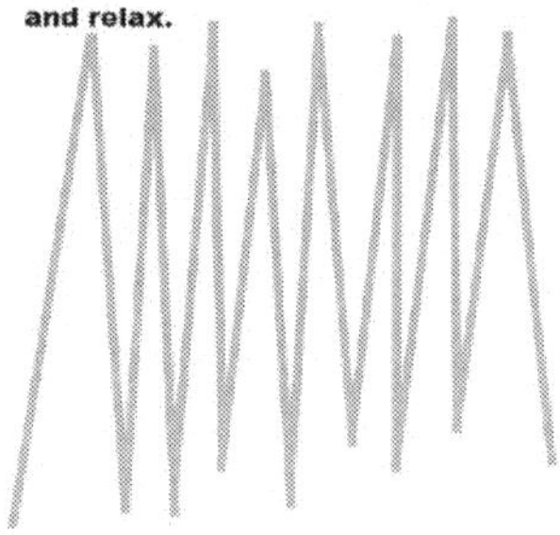

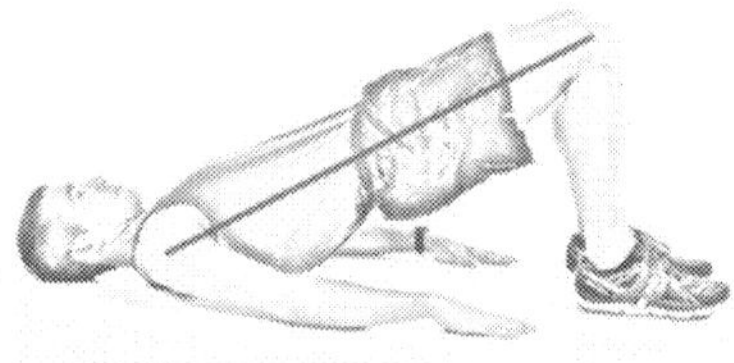

Finally, as you exhale press your feet into the floor, slowly lift your pelvis up off the mat into a bridge, your pelvis is in line with your shoulders and knees, hold this position for 10 seconds. Remember to breathe! Release and roll slowly back down to the floor.

**If you cannot hold this position, as an alternative you can place a cushion under your buttocks to keep them raised,*

In the first 2 weeks:

Hold the squeeze for a count of 6 and take a break before to continue the exercise for a count of 5. Before repeating the exercise (Part A-B), take a break counting to 30. Repeat the exercise 3 times.

Between 2 - 4 weeks:

Hold the squeeze for a count of 8 and take a break before to continue the exercise for a count of 5. Before repeating the exercise, take a break counting to 30. Repeat the exercise 4 times.

After 4 weeks:

Hold the squeeze for a count of 10 and take a break before to continue the exercise for a count of 5. Before repeating the exercise, take a break counting to 30. Repeat the exercise 5 times.

“Bow Tie” exercise:

Sit in "Z" leg position (the legs make the shape of a letter “Z”); the left knee pulled up in front and the right heel pulled back. Relax your abdominal muscles.

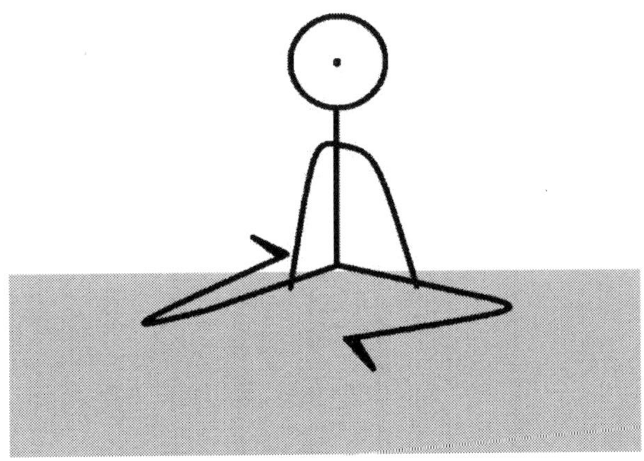

**If you are not able to settle yourself in this Z-leg position you can sit in butterfly position.*

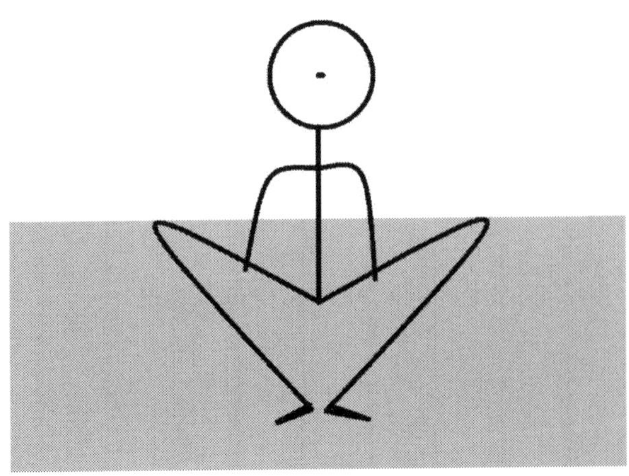

Sit with your soles of your feet together, so in this position your knees point out to the sides. Grab your legs with your hands.

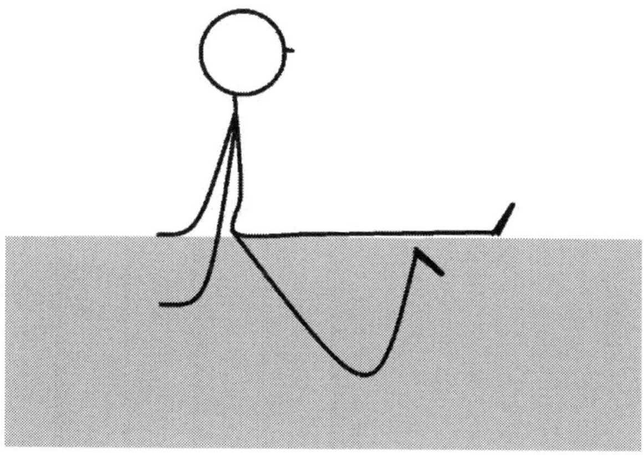

**Another alternative position, Open your legs wide as you can, in the shape of the letter V, then, bend your right knee and place the sole of your left foot beside to the left knee, change the direction with the legs.*

The task is to perform gradually a Control Total squeeze counting to 4, hold the squeeze for a count of 6, without relaxing the muscles, immediately perform 4 Control Total contractions, as quickly as you can, increase again the strength of the contraction till your maximum force and at the and counting to 4, gradually let your pelvic floor muscles completely relax. Before repeating the exercise, take a break counting to 30.

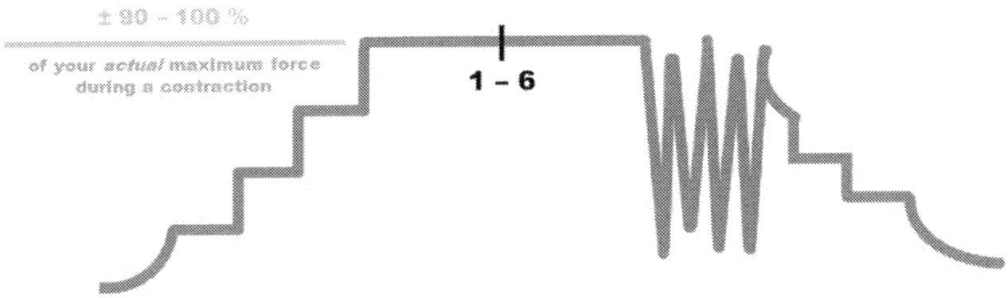

In the first 2 weeks:

Hold the squeeze for a count of 6. Before repeating the exercise, take a break counting to 30. Repeat the exercise 3 times. Change the direction with the legs (by the position 1 or 3)

Between 2 - 4 weeks:

Hold the squeeze for a count of 10. Before repeating the exercise, take a break counting to 30. Repeat the exercise 4 times.

After 4 weeks:

Hold the squeeze for a count of 12. Before repeating the exercise, take a break counting to 30. Repeat the exercise 5 times.

Penis power exercise:

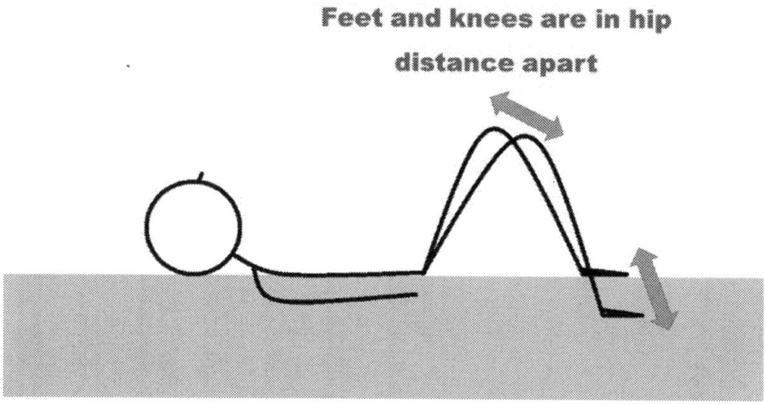

In supine position with knees bent, feet flat on the floor. Feet and knees are in hip distance apart. The task is to perform suddenly a contraction with the muscles around and in the penis, up to the 50% of the maximum strength, right after increase the force of the squeeze up to your maximum force, then perform 4 short and fast contraction but releasing back the strength of the squeeze only up to the 50 % of your maximum force, after increase again and hold the squeeze on the maximum strength counting to 6. Release the contraction of the muscles back only up to the 50 % of your maximum force - hold the squeeze at 50% counting to 4 at the and gradually let the muscles to relax completely. Exhale slowly.

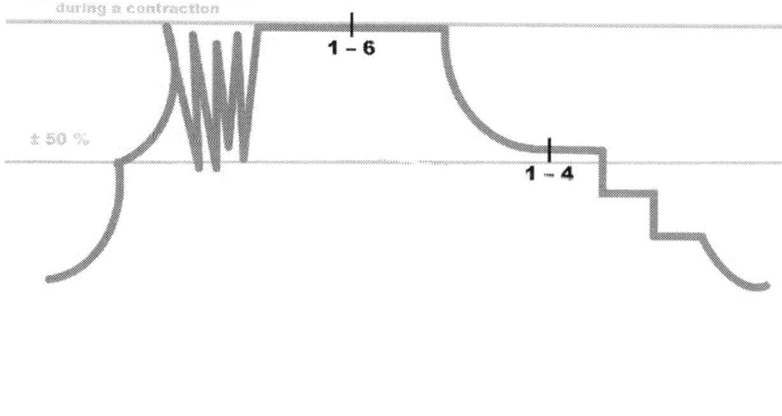

In the first 2 weeks:

Hold the squeeze at the maximum force for a count of 6 and on the 50% of the maximum force counting to 4. Before repeating the exercise, take a break counting to 30. Repeat the exercise 3 times.

Between 2-4 weeks:

Hold the squeeze at the maximum force for a count of 8 and on the 50% of the maximum force counting to 6. Before repeating the exercise, take a break counting to 30. Repeat the exercise 4 times.

After 4 weeks:

Hold the squeeze at the maximum force for a count of 10 and on the 50% of the maximum force counting to 10. Before repeating the exercise, take a break counting to 30. Repeat the exercise 4 times.

At the end of the repetitions of the exercise, one time, perform 8 definite, short, fast and strong contraction with the muscles around and in your penis; as quickly as you can. Do not try to hold on to the contractions; just squeeze and relax. Remain in supine position, with knees bent. Feet and knees are very close to each other or closed. In order to maintain a balance, place your arms on the floor alongside your body, palms facing down. As you exhale press your feet into the floor, slowly lift your pelvis up off the mat into a bridge, your pelvis is in line with your shoulders and knees, hold this position for 10 seconds. Remember to breathe! Release and roll slowly back down to the floor. Inhale deeply through your nose into your abdomen and slowly blow out the air while you relax your pelvis completely.

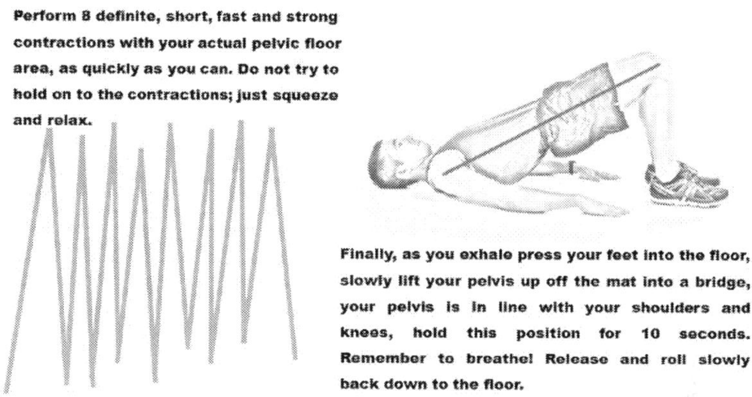

Exercise to strengthen the anal sphincter:

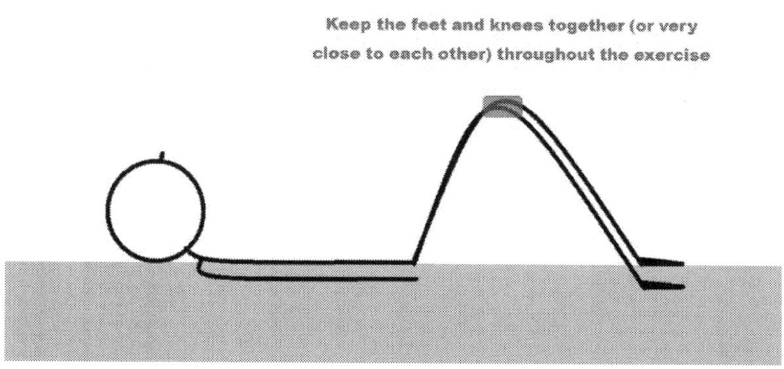

In supine position, keep the feet and knees together or very close to each other.

The task is, meantime you count to 4, gradually squeeze the anal sphincter muscle till the maximum of your force, hold the contraction on the 100% for a count of 4, relax the muscles around the anus up to 50% of the maximum strength and hold the squeeze on 50% for a count of 4, increase again the force of the contraction till your maximum force and hold the squeeze on the 100% for a count of 4, at the and meantime you count to 4, gradually relax your anal sphincter muscle. Exhale slowly.

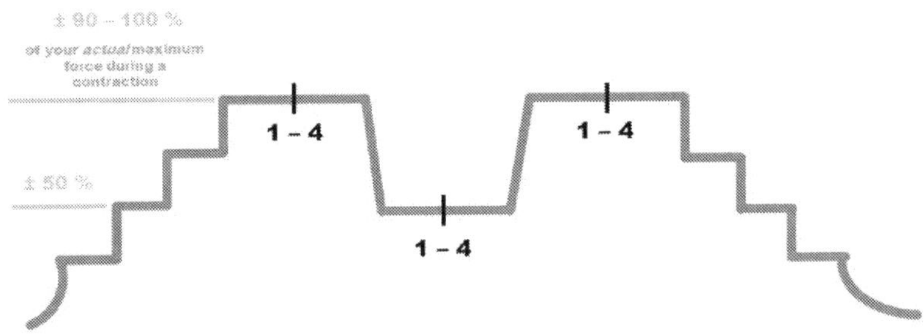

In the first 2 weeks:

Hold the squeeze at the maximum force for a count of 4 - on the 50% of the maximum force counting to 4 - at the maximum force again for a count of 4. Before repeating the exercise, take a break counting to 30. Repeat the exercise 3 times.

Between 2-4 weeks:

Hold the squeeze at the maximum force for a count of 6 - on the 50% of the maximum force counting to 6 - at the maximum force again for a count of 6. Before repeating the exercise, take a break counting to 30. Repeat the exercise 4 times.

After 4 weeks:

Hold the squeeze at the maximum force for a count of 10 - on the 50% of the maximum force counting to 6 - at the maximum force again for a count of 10. Before repeating the exercise, take a break counting to 30. Repeat the exercise 5 times.

At the end of the repetition of the exercise, one time, perform 8 definite, short, fast and strong contraction with the anal sphincter muscle, as quickly as you can. Do not try to hold on the contractions; just squeeze and relax. Remain in supine position, with knees bent. Feet and knees are very close to each other or closed. In order to maintain a balance, place your arms on the floor alongside your body, palms facing down. As you exhale press your feet into the floor, slowly lift your pelvis up off the mat into a bridge, your pelvis is in line with your shoulders and knees; hold this position for 10 seconds. Remember to breathe! Release and roll slowly back down to the floor. Inhale deeply through your nose into your abdomen and slowly blow out the air while you relax your pelvis completely.

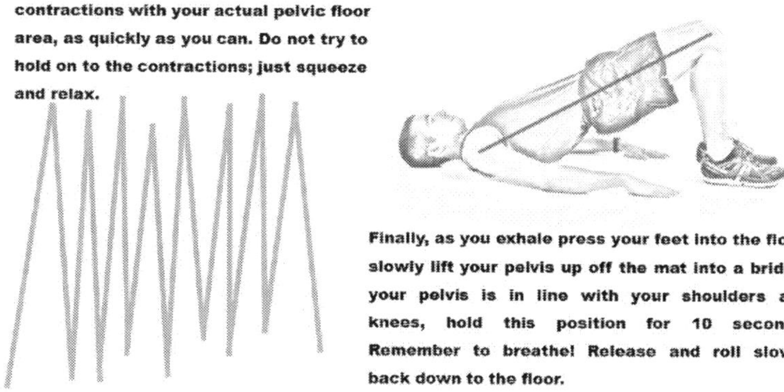

Total pelvic power exercise

In the following 3 postures:

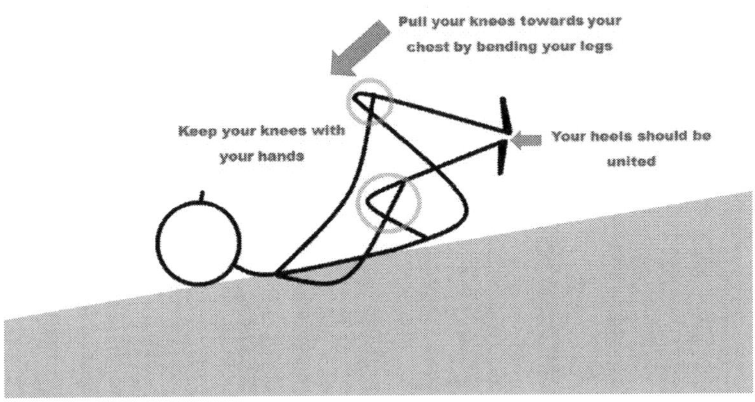

Lying position. Pull both knees toward your chest by flexing your legs. Keep your knees with your hands. Your heels should be united.

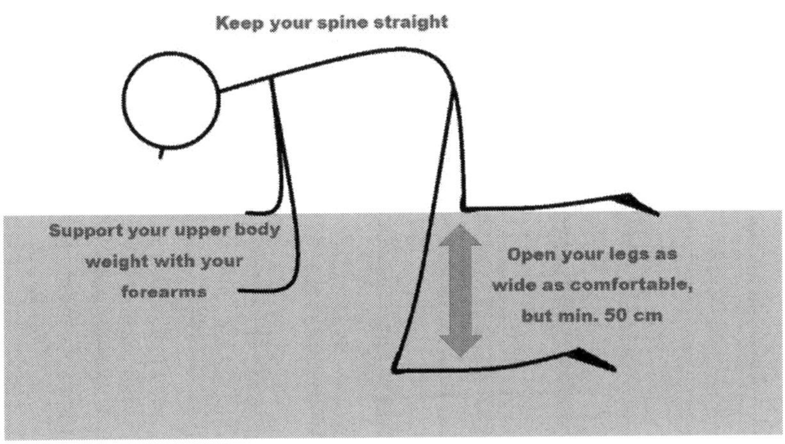

In "all fours" position. Support your upper - body weight with your forearms. Keep your spine straight. Open your legs as wide as comfortable but min. should be 50 cm.

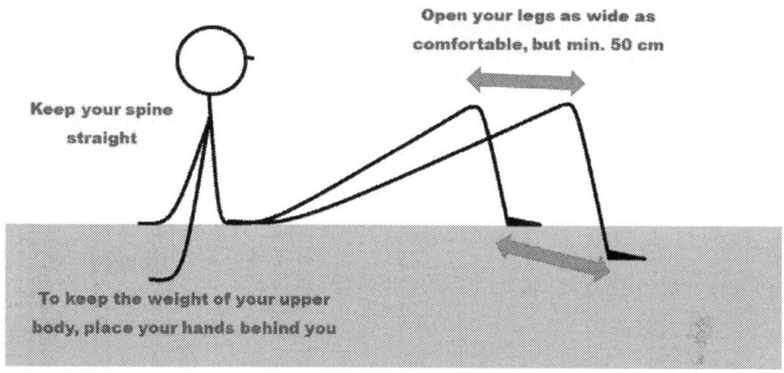

In sitting position with knees bent. Keep your spine straight. Support your upper body with your hands. Spread your legs as wide apart as you can.

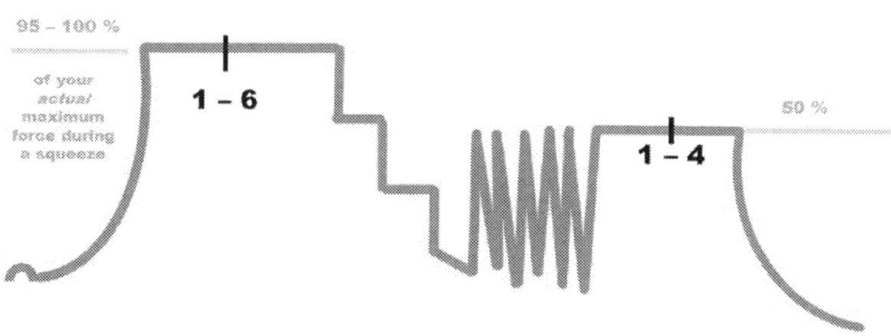

The task is to perform suddenly a Control Total squeeze up to the maximum force, hold the squeeze for a count of 6, then gradually counting to 4, let the pelvic floor muscles to relax, right after perform 6 Control Total squeeze as quickly as you can, without a break, perform suddenly again a Control Total contraction up to the 50 % of your maximum force, hold the squeeze for a count of 4, at the end let your pelvic floor muscles completely to relax.

In the first 4 weeks:

Hold the squeeze at the maximum of your force as you count to 6 - on the 50% of the maximum strength counting to 4. Before repeating the exercise, take a break counting to 30. Repeat the exercise 2 times in each postures.

After 4 weeks:

Hold the squeeze at the maximum force for a count of 10 - on the 50% of the maximum force counting to 10. Before repeating the exercise, take a break counting to 30. Repeat the exercise 2 times in each postures.

A final word

Real success will only be achieved by the application of this method, if you do these exercises on a regular basis. 15 minutes of exercise per day or at least 3 times a week will be essential to reach the goal, to strengthen pelvic floor muscles. Practicing is the indispensable key to success. The result depends on how can you insert the set of exercises of the training in your daily schedule on a regular basis, and how can you apply the useful advices of the IWT® program in your everyday life. If you abandon the training, your muscles will weaken again. This is a program for life; it should be part of your daily routine like washing your teeth regularly. If you repeatedly delay or put the exercise off, always finding an excuse, it actually proves that you are not important enough for yourself.

Well, I have tried to summarize just the most important pieces of information. They can be applied by anyone, starting even right now.

Let us treat our body and health as a value to be preserved in the long run, being responsible for it ourselves.

I wish you much success in doing so in the future!

Congratulations on starting your journey to good Sexual Health!

GLOSSARY

Anal sphincters: two rings of muscles surrounding the rectum and anus, which help to control passage of bowel movements.

Anus: the final two inches of rectum, surrounded by the internal and external anal sphincter muscle, is the outlet for solid waste (stool).

Bacteria: microscopic one-celled plants. Some bacteria are harmless or even beneficial; others can cause infection. Most prostate infections are caused by common forms of bacteria found in the gastrointestinal system.

Benign Prostatic Hyperplasia (BPH): condition characterized by growth of a benign tumor inside the prostate, often resulting in voiding difficulties, also known as benign prostate hypertrophy.

Bladder: the bladder is a stretchable, muscular organ located inside the pelvic cavity, it is supported by the pelvic floor muscles, retains urine until it is excreted from the body.

Bowel movement: the act of passing feces (stool) through the anus.

Bowels: another word for intestines or colon.

Bulbocavernosus muscle: in males, encircles the bulb or root of the penis and conncets it to the perineal body. In the daily life plays an important role in the mechanism of voluntary urination, when we want to start or stop the flow of urine. In addition, helps empty the urethra at the end of urination and expels semen during ejaculation.

Calculus: hardened, stonelike mass of high calcium content sometimes formed in the kidney, bladder and prostate. Prostate stones are generally not dangerous, but influencing negatively its normal function, may contribute to chronic prostatitis or in several cases to prostate cancer.

Catheter: A narrow flexible tube that is inserted into the urethra and the bladder for the purpose of draining urine.

Chronic prostatitis: persistent form of prostatitis, lasting for an extended period- sometimes years.

Colon: lower section of the large intestine leading into the rectum.

Constipation: a condition in which bowel movements are less frequent than normal, hard, dry and firm bowel movements, the evacuation of feces is difficult and infrequent.

Continence: the ability to exercise voluntary control over the urge, to void urinate or defecate or passing gas, until an appropriate time and place.

Contraindication: side effects of a (medical) treatment which would indicate the treatment is more harmful than the indeed benefits.

Cystitis: inflammation of the bladder, usually caused by an infection.

Cystoscopy: diagnostic procedure for urological examination allowing viewing inside the urethra and bladder.

Defecate: the act of having a bowel movement.

Dehydration: a state that occurs when not enough fluid is present to fulfill the body's fluid needs.

Diuretic: any drug, beverage or food that promotes increased urine excretion.

Ejaculation: ejection of sperm and seminal fluid from the penis from contraction of muscles in the urethra and prostate area.

Epididymis: two common-shaped tubes inside the scrotum that that surround and holds the testicles in place.

Estrogen: one of the most important sex hormones, contributing to development of female sex characteristics, regulates sexual organs and their functions.

Evacuation: another word for a bowel movement.

External sphincter: the outer layer of the sphincter muscle, usually under voluntary control.

Fecal incontinence: the accidental and involuntary loss of fecal material (stool) of gas from the anus.

Feces (stool): waste material produced from the intestines. Feces are produced of bacteria, undigested food and material produced the intestines.

Flatulence: the release of gas through the anus.

Fungal infection: infection of prostate or another part of the body caused by a fungus microorganism such as candida.

Gas: material that results from swallowed air or produced from certain foods or that is created when bacteria in the colon break down waste material.

Impotence: inability of a man to achieve or maintain an erection of sufficient duration to satisfy both sexual partners.

Incontinence: inability to retain urine within the bladder or feces within the colon. Incontinence among men may be complete or partial and can result from prostate surgery of from radiation therapy for prostate cancer.

Internal sphincter: the internal layer of the sphincter muscle, usually under involuntary control.

Intra-abdominal: inside the abdominal cavity.

Kegel exercises: exercises with repetitive contractions of the PC muscles; used to strengthen pelvic floor muscles or to decrease or eliminate incontinence, erection problems other inconvenient intimate problems. Kegel exercises may help to prevent or eliminate incontinence following prostate surgery.

Kidneys: two parallel glandular organs that continually filter the blood to separate waste products from the blood.

Levator ani: the main muscle of the pelvic floor, made up of different parts.

Lower back pain: pain in the lower region of the back which frequently is due to a prostate disorder.

Magnesium: metallic mineral essential in the diets. Magnesium may play a special role in prostate health.

Orchiectomy: surgical removal of one or both testicles.

Overflow incontinence: The involuntary loss of urine, associated with over distension of the bladder.

Pelvic floor: the muscle floor of the abdominal cavity, supports the pelvic organs.

Pelvic floor muscles: a small band of muscle below the pelvic organs, normally assists in maintaining continence.

Pelvic organ prolapse: a condition in which one or more organs and connective tissues within the pelvic cavity shift in a downward direction out of their normal anatomical position.

Penis: the male organ used for urination.

Perineum: area of muscle and tissue between the scrotum and anus.

Premature ejaculation: male sexual dysfunction when ejaculation occurs well before desired by both partners, may be caused also by prostatitis.

Prostate: firm, muscular gland in males that surrounds the urethra near the outlet of the bladder.

Prostate massage: stroking and kneading the prostate using a gloved finger inserted through the rectum. Prostate massage is used to relive prostate congestion (painful buildup of prostatic fluid in the prostate) or obtain a sample of prostatic fluid for laboratory examination.

Prostatectomy: surgical removal of all or part of the prostate gland.

Prostatitis: infection of the prostate caused usually by bacteria; can be acute or chronic.

Pubic bone: lower front part of the pelvis.

Pubic symphysis: where the two pubic bones meet.

Pubococcygeus or PC muscle: PC muscles the muscle that supports the organs and tissues of the pelvic region. Kegel exercises are designed to strengthen these muscles and may help to alleviate incontinence, prolapse or hemorrhoid problems in men and women.

Pudendal nerves: innervates the external urethral and anal sphincters and the pelvic and urogenital diaphragm muscles; it is part of the voluntary nervous system.

Radical prostatectomy: complete removal of the prostate gland, to treat prostate cancer.

Rectocele: prolapse in which the anterior or posterior rectal wall bulges forward or posteriorly. In males may also develop a rectocele but rarely.

Rectum: last several inches of the intestines; the lowest part of the bowel found just above the anus.

Reflex incontinence: loss of urine due to the hyperactivity of the bladder muscle and / or involuntary urethral relaxation in the absence of the sensation associated with the desire to urinate.

Risk factor: quality that makes a person more susceptible to a specific disease.

Scrotum: external pouch of skin containing the testicles and epididymis.

Sphincter: group of circular muscles, surrounding an opening in the body that tightens and relaxes to control the flow of fluid through the opening. There are internal and external urethral and anal sphincters.

Stress incontinence: a form of urinary incontinence characterized by the involuntary small loss of urine with increased intra-abdominal pressure during physical exertion: for example during; coughing, sneezing, laughing, jumping, running.

Testicles: two glands located inside the scrotum that produce sperm and sex hormones including testosterone.

Testosterone: principal male sex hormone that is responsible for male sexual characteristic as well as the growth of benign and malignant prostatic tissue.

Urethra: a muscular tube, which is connecting the bladder to the outside, carries urine away from the bladder.

Urge incontinence: Urinary incontinence, sudden leaking of relatively large amounts of urine when the bladder muscle involuntarily contracts.

Urinary incontinence: loss of control over urinary storage function, thus leakage of urine.

Urinary retention: quantities of urine backing up in the bladder which can cause bladder and kidney damage.

Urologist: physician specializing in disorders of the urinary system.

Vaginal yeast infection: Vaginal infection in women caused by microscopic yeast organisms. Yeast infections can be sexually transmitted and can cause a form of prostatitis.

Voluntary control: conscious control.

Zinc: metallic mineral essential in the diets of humans. Normally, the prostate contains a high concentration of zinc, so there is a good evidence that zinc is important to prostate health.

Printed in Great Britain
by Amazon

48576981R00087